THE 5 PRINCIPLES

A REVOLUTIONARY PATH TO HEALTH, INNER WEALTH, AND KNOWLEDGE OF SELF

KHNUM "STIC" IBOMU

balance

New York   Boston

Balance
Hachette Book Group
1290 Avenue of the Americas, New York, NY 10104
grandcentralpublishing.com
twitter.com/grandcentralpub

First edition: October 2022

Balance is an imprint of Grand Central Publishing. The Balance name and logo are trademarks of Hachette Book Group, Inc.

The publisher is not responsible for websites (or their content) that are not owned by the publisher.

Library of Congress Control Number: 2022940002

ISBNs: 9781538708088 (hardcover), 978153870810¹ (ebook)

Printed in the United States of America

LSC-C

Printing 1, 2022

Contents

Contents

A Note from the Author: Native Tongue

I've been an emcee since fifth grade. Communicating with words is an art form that I have practiced for nearly five decades and one that I greatly respect.

With that in mind, I decided to write this book in my native tongue. What I mean by that is: It's gonna be in my true voice. It's gonna be a mix of Ebonics, some country Shadeville, Florida, twang from where I was born and raised, some up-top Brooklyn slang from where I came of age, and then at other times I'mma be nerding out and diving deep into philosophical concepts and introducing ideas and words that might be new to you. I might bust into rap lyrics or quote anybody from rappers to swamis, from athletes to activists, from gangstas to gurus, because all of these influences are part of my authentic voice—that's me, that's who I am, and that's how I talk, and I wanted to just be myself and tell my story and share the game I've picked up on my journey authentically and comfortably.

Participles are gonna be dangling all over this motherfucker, so if you're a stickler for standard grammar, this ain't that book. My bad in advance. It's more natural, authentic, and honest for me to write in my everyday conversational flow; and plus I knew I was gonna do an audio version and so I wanted it to sound like it's actually my voice and my style of communication, not some textbook-sounding shit.

And trust me, I started writing at first in that super academic *poindexter* voice in my head, the one that's like those super critical

English teachers who think the only way to articulate well is to edit out all the shit that makes language fresh and interesting—no Black vernacular, no "ain't finta be this" or "gon' be that." And why not?

Don't get me wrong, I love great writing whether it be formal or colloquial. What I started with was very formal—and it was my story, and it was what I was trying to say, but it ain't feel like *me* saying it. It ain't have the *feeling*. It was too sterile and too stiff, so I scrapped it and started all over again. I believe language should serve us, not the other way around.

There is a place for formal standard English, like academic spaces where that is a requirement, and then there is a place where you just kick back and be you, like when speaking with close friends. So that's the vibe I wanted for this book: one friend chopping it up with another, ya dig? In hip-hop we bilingual anyway. If you can relate and resonate with hip-hop, you'll be able to pick up what I'm dropping.

Introduction

This is your life. How you live it is up to you.

But the truth is, it ain't gonna last forever, and as we age, things are going to get more challenging healthwise, like it or not. How we take care of ourselves now will likely be the biggest determining factor in how well we age. The stress we carry, the unhealthy foods we binge on, the toxic substances we party with, the workouts we skip, the breaks we didn't take, and the lack of healthy disciplines in our lives all come with a price. Every unhealthy choice we make adds on to that tab until one day, it's time to pay up.

The average life span in the US is about seventy-nine years. I think that number is well below what could be possible with a holistic and healthy lifestyle, but based on how the average person is living, those are the numbers, and the numbers don't lie. But even for those who make it to seventy-nine years, how many of those years are lived in vibrant health? People are being diagnosed younger and younger with all sorts of preventable diseases and conditions.

I want to acknowledge those sad stats, but I promise you this ain't a book based on fear and scare tactics. Not at all. We all presumably want to live a long, healthy, and meaningful life, right? The bad news is that nobody can predict the future, but the great news is there are some very, very simple principles and practices that we can implement in our lives to help us thrive. This is a book about the positive and revolutionary effects of a healthy lifestyle. This is not a book about what the physical body looks like or this trending diet versus that diet, this book is about the journey of well-rounded well-being.

Even though my day job for the last couple decades has been a hip-hop artist and producer with dead prez, a lot of people may not know I'm a certified long-distance running coach and a longtime student of the martial arts, or why and how I became so passionate about health and fitness in the first place. The many disciplines I talk about at length in the chapters to come have revolutionized my health, fitness, mindset, and life. But even more importantly, I wanted to take my personal transformation and all my experiences in martial arts, running, plant-based nutrition, meditation, and more and break them down into a gang of actionable takeaways for you to get your own personal benefits from them. You don't have to be a martial artist or a runner to benefit, and you don't have to be perfect—I'm sure not. You just have to stay focused. Focus is one of my strengths, and I believe these principles can deeply inspire you to focus on your well-being on a whole new level. And hopefully what we heal in our own selves, we'll heal in the family tree to come as well.

The World Health Organization defines health as "a state of complete physical, mental and social well-being and not merely the absence of disease or sickness," and that's right in alignment with what my experience, experiments, and being a guinea pig for a nutritionist and holistic health counselor for almost thirty years have taught me. You especially see this when you start taking care of elders in your family as early as in their sixties, struggling with preventable health issues. When you see how quickly poor lifestyle habits develop into chronic illness, it gives you perspective. It ain't gotta be like that. The medical system got drugs to treat the symptoms, but then you need drugs for the side effects of the drugs, and before you know it, your organs, your kidneys and liver, are destroyed. What is the cure? That old adage is true: an ounce of prevention beats a pound of cure. Living a long time is one thing, but living those years vibrantly well, that's the real goal. I see it like this: if it's in the master plan for my life, I'mma do all I can to be thriving, naturally, into the triple digits!

So dig, if you're searching for less stress in your life and more peace of mind (ain't we all?), if you are striving to eat better but don't know what to trust, if you know you need to exercise more but haven't found the right fit to make fitness a part of your lifestyle, if you are a workaholic who don't know how to allow yourself time to rest, or if you are someone who feels like you just lack the drive to stay disciplined to make healthy choices and do the healthy things in your best interest, *The 5 Principles* is definitely the right book, at the right time, for you.

Over the eighty thousand some odd words of this book, with lots of self-reflection and a tremendous amount of support from my literary agency, Serendipity; my publisher, Balance (shout-out Regina, Kelly, Nana, and the whole team); and my friends and family who listened and gave constructive feedback, I've been able to organize the jewels from my journey and lifestyle into this book: the wellness principles that I strive to live by and have come to thrive by over the last couple decades.

The 5 Principles is kind of a hybrid type of book. It's part memoir, in that I share personal stories from my health and fitness journey. It's part manifesto, in that we explore inspiring philosophies and revolutionary ideas that empower well-being. And part manual, as it's full of practices and actionable takeaways, tips, and techniques that you can try on for size.

We explore everything from why the right mindset matters, to listening to your own gut about nutrition, to finding your fitness, to prioritizing self-care and respecting rest, to staying motivated and consistent. It's not about just knowing health facts, it's about embracing how to actually enjoy the discipline.

So, if you're into hanging out with a rapper for a little while who is passionate about all things well-being, and you're ready to be inspired by real-life practices that have really changed the game for me and others, with no further ado, let's get it.

—*Stic*

MINDSET MATTERS

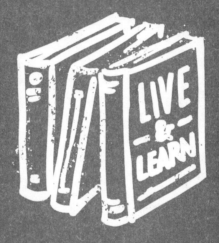

CHAPTER 1

Unlearn

It was '93. I was around nineteen or so, living in my hometown of Tallahassee, Florida. The streetlights were just starting to glow. I was sitting at the top of the stairwell outside the door of our little hustle spot in the hood on the corner of Holton Street and Osceola when a silver car I didn't recognize pulled up. I kept my strategic distance at the top of the stairs instead of going down to meet them. The bearded dude in the driver's seat started yelling up to me, talking real greasy and asking where one of my homeboys was, cursing and making threats about what he was going to do when he found him. I had become a hard shell in those days, and I didn't give a fuck about much. I always kept a pistol on me, and as he was mouthing off, I started thinking to myself, This dude got some nerve to pull up to our spot making threats. How he think we the type of folk you can just run up on like that?

Not on my watch.

Blam! Blam! Blam!

I hadn't even given it much thought. It was a street code and I had embraced it: bomb first. You can't let dudes think they can run over you. You have to let 'em know it ain't sweet, so I made the first move. Dude mashed the gas and sped off so fast in the car he almost crashed into the stop sign turning the corner. It happened so quickly; I didn't even know where my shots landed. It was getting dark and harder to see clearly, but I noticed across the street there was someone laying out in the parking lot, which was a normal thing over there but for a moment I wondered if I had accidentally struck him or if he had already been there.

I didn't even bother to check. In my mind at that time, I was a soldier in those streets, and all I knew was if I felt like I needed to protect mine, busting my gun was just part of the protocol.

I stuck my pistol back in the waistline of my khakis and calmly walked back inside our spot, closed the door, and sat down on the couch like nothing happened.

My homey who was also there was heated.

"Dawg, what the fuck? What did you do that for?" he asked.

"This sucker was talking shit and I wasn't going for it. It ain't nothing," I said nonchalantly.

My boy already sensed what I was too oblivious to realize: reckless gunplay like that was only going to attract unwanted attention. I was so clueless I couldn't even see what would come next.

Boom, boom, boom.

"TPD! Open up!!!" The pounding got louder.

Boom! Boom! Boom!

"Tallahassee Police Department. Open up, now!!!"

Oh shit! Police at the door? I got this hot pistol on me. We had all these little plastic baggies of herb spread all over the bed in the back room that my boy rushed to try and hide. There was no back door for escape and no time to jump out of a window. My homeboy stashed the weed as best he could, and I hid the .38 in the couch cushions. The cops were banging on the door, and I knew if I didn't open the door fast, they were going to kick it in or start shooting. Just as I went to open the door, four cops rushed in like linebackers yelling, "Get down! Get down!" One of the cops gun-butted me on the forehead; I was tackled to the floor onto my chest and put in cuffs.

I went to jail that night.

But hold that thought. We'll come back to that in a sec.

As I reflect on that troubling time in my life with you now, almost thirty years later, it's safe to say the journey between then and now has been nothing short of revolutionary! Being just a few years away from fifty, I'm reminded of one of my favorite quotes from one of my favorite icons, Muhammad Ali: "The man who views the world at fifty the same as he did at twenty has wasted thirty years of his life." It's crazy thinking about how far I've come as a man from the frustrated kid that I was at that time. I have been truly blessed to travel the world with my rap group dead prez and experience all the life-changing cultural blessings and commercial accolades that have come with being a successful hip-hop artist.

We've released our own classic albums and songs, and I've also written, produced, collaborated, and toured with some of the best of the best, from Nas to Jay-Z to Erykah Badu, The Roots, Kanye West, and many others. I've also been on the front lines of community causes dear to my heart: raising awareness about police brutality, supporting political prisoner campaigns, and lending energy of solidarity to grassroots initiatives for change around the world. I've released two number-one albums in the "fit-hop" genre that I invented, *The Workout* and *Workout II*, and I'm still only just beginning to break ground on the mountains of synergy between hip-hop and healthy living.

I've received awards and critical acclaim for my work as a hip-hop artist and as an activist and advocate. I've also developed powerful partnerships with some of the biggest brands in the world as a creative director. I'm an entrepreneur, an author, a certified long-distance running coach, a longtime student of the martial arts, an archery instructor, and at the time of this writing, I'm also an adjunct professor at New York University. My path has taken me from being a youth full of rage to becoming a father of two amazing sons. I'm healthy, enjoying life, and grateful.

I don't say all of that to flex, but to give you a real sense of just how much impact the five principles that I'll share in this book have had on my life and overall well-being. The five Ps, as I like to call them, are fundamental truths that form the cornerstones of my well-being, because they have not only improved my mental and physical health and fitness, but they've helped me grow spiritually and continue to help me evolve as a person.

I definitely didn't start out on a healthy path, and maybe you ain't on one right now either, or maybe you are. Either way, I want you to know that I learned to value these principles by how they've impacted my life for the better, and I'm sharing them with you because I know they will make a profound difference in your life no matter who you are, where you are from, or where you're at right now. And that's on everything I love. If you're already on your healthy gangsta flex, I'mma give you some ways to mix it up and keep it going. If you're just stepping into your wellness journey, you're gonna get a solid road map for a healthy lifestyle, tailor-fit to who you are, that flows with your unique goals as you go and grow. You don't have to be perfect, but you do have to be focused.

Before I get ahead of myself, let's get back to the focus at hand. Where was I? Oh right, in Leon County Jail.

Me Time

Time in a cell can be a game changer,
I can hate it or redirect that same anger
Get focused on life like in a monk's chamber
Get physically fit back on my healthy gangsta.
—"Me Time" by Stic, *Workout II*

One thing about jail is that it forces you to sit down. Being still can provide its own medicine. One day during my incarceration I was daydreaming, sitting down on the edge of my bunk in my "county blues" uniform staring at the concrete cell floor, and somehow I slipped out of my normal state of consciousness and into a sort of trance. The best way to describe it is that my mind—or my mind's eye—was looking out of the front windshield of a car onto a road but there was no car, and the road seemed to be just arising out of nowhere as I explored around. Was I going crazy? It felt like my mind was watching something happen, but I also had the sense that I was somehow creating the road ahead of me at the same time. Was I choosing this or was my mind choosing it? The power of that question in itself made me start to consider, what is the distinction between "me" and "my mind"? I decided to test what was happening. I thought "right," and the road curved to the right. I formed the intention of "left" and sure enough, things swerved left. I kept on down the road like this. I still wasn't sure what the hell I was experiencing so to test the possibilities even more, I had the random idea of candy canes popping out of the ground like telegraph poles. As soon as I had the thought, boom—red-and-white candy canes appeared out of nowhere. All this time I was in this trance state, I was oblivious to everything else— my focus and attention were completely absorbed in the moment; the experience had arisen by itself and I was just flowing along with this wild ride inside my mind, in awe. But then, all of a sudden, I snapped out of it when I thought to myself, Whoa, I must be hallucinating. Did these jail motherfuckers try to poison me with the water or the food I ate? Am I going crazy? I was back in the reality of sitting on the edge of my bed in that concrete cell just like that.

The entire experience lasted probably less than ten minutes, but for those lucid moments, dog, I was somewhere else. It's like I had escaped from jail and I was free on a whole other level. I didn't understand what had happened, but the quality of those minutes opened something inside of me. It showed me that there are way more levels of the mind to explore beyond the everyday thoughts and worries and noise floating around in our heads. For just a brief moment in time, I had found a path in my own mind to leave that jail and be free. It was like my subconscious mind was showing me that through my conscious choices, I have the power to create the road ahead of me in my real life. They had my body. But they couldn't lock my mind down.

It wasn't the first time I'd been to jail, but it was the first time I had been in jail for months at a time. I remember just looking around in the dormitory and really taking in just how many generations of us were in there—the whole spectrum of us on lockdown: from the young and don't give a fuck like I was at the time to gray-hair OGs that still didn't give a fuck. It was straight bros, gay cats, geniuses, the mentally challenged, dudes in lockup for traffic violations, probation violations, scams, domestic violence, drug possession, Muslims, Christians, college kids, and plenty of cats swearing their innocence—every type of individual you can imagine. No matter what side of the track, we were all packed in that motherfucker together. It felt like a human penalty box we'd all somehow ended up in from the circumstances and conditions that set up the choices we'd made in our lives. I was like, Damn, I fell for the trap, too! I was starting to see the game for what it is and coming to grips with the very likely possibility that if I didn't make some changes in the street life mentality I was trapped in, I'd be another statistic coming in and out of jail for the rest of my life or worse.

It was the wake-up call I needed.

Shifting My Mindset

Time stands still in jail, and you don't get let out just because you feel like you've learned your lesson. I still had to sit down for the rest of my sentence even though my spirit was ready to leap out them gates. I worked in the kitchen two times a day, serving the county slop they called food and cleaning off trays after feed time was over. The work was monotonous, but it got me out of my cell twice a day and it helped pass the time. More than anything though, I was reading my ass off. Jail staff brought carts full of books once a week, and I was grabbing everything I could. I really got into one giant book called *Dianetics*, which, I found out much later, was authored by L. Ron Hubbard, who had his own share of controversies, but that's another story. At the time, the book was right on time for me and very enlightening. It went deep into theories on philosophy and the mind, different aspects of how the brain works, how the way we perceive things can be influenced and manipulated, and how trauma and negative behaviors from the past show up in our choices and experiences. As I thought about those insights applied to my own life, I started realizing more and more how the survival-mode mentality I had learned on the block was actually blocking my progress. At times I played cards with the other guys and I picked up drawing again, a hobby I had as a youth, but more than anything I was reading about the mind and self-reflecting every chance I got.

My mindset was slowly shifting, but I still had a long way to go before I'd shake a lot more shackles and unhealthy habits I picked up in the streets. My mom and dad visited me on two separate occasions, and I apologized for my actions to them both and let them know I was planning on making better choices. They were disappointed but supportive and encouraging. My lady Afya was showing me she was a rider; even though we'd only just been together for some months at that time, she visited me every single day I was incarcerated. That meant a lot to me. Other inmates were jealous and made jokes every time I'd get called on for another visit, but I didn't care what they thought. Those visits from my mom and pops and seeing Afya show up consistently, making the effort to come and support me, helped me start to recognize how much my life and choices mattered not only to myself, but to people I cared about most: my family and community.

I thought a lot about the different positive and negative influences I'd had in my life up to that point—the foundations I'd learned at home, the many explicit and implicit lessons I learned there, where I aligned and where I didn't. I questioned religion. I question everything. I thought about all of the seeds that had been planted in my dome by so many diverse sectors of my surrounding community. I had received a kind of diplomatic immunity in so many circles, as the young rap dude who was kicked out of a racist high school that everyone wanted to look out for and offer their mentorship to help me grow and stay out of trouble. I thought about how I had veered off the path of all my early culturally conscious influences and how the ideas I picked up in the streets about what being a G meant had become a hardwired part of my mentality. I reflected on all the Afrocentric mentors around town that had embraced me and let me crash on their couches and taught me about our culture and allowed me to soak up their knowledge. I'll get into this more in Chapter 3, but being a local hanging on and around the HBCU Florida Agricultural and Mechanical University (FAMU) campus, though I never enrolled, had given me a positive education in a gang of ways. Although I had fallen for a lot of the traps in the streets that I'd already been made aware were out there, all those powerful seeds were not wasted on me. They just took their time to sprout.

The Trap

Black lives matter, fasho. All lives matter fasho. But to borrow a phrase from Oprah—you know how she always says "What I know for sure"—I can say this: *as a Black man and as a human being*, what I know fasho, so much so that it's literally principle number one in my book, is *mindset* matters.

Mindset is the outlook, perspective, level of self-awareness, and mental filter that we make our choices through, and it matters in so many ways to the success of anything we want to be, do, or have in life. I saw an interview where the late, great poet Gil Scott-Heron was explaining the meaning behind his classic masterpiece *"The*

Revolution Will Not Be Televised." He said the most significant revolution can't be viewed on television because that revolution happens in your mind.

I wasn't in my right mind when I fired those shots that landed me in the county jail. Shit, I was so hardheaded at that time I didn't know what my right mind even was. Before I could ever even think about getting to the point where the knucklehead I was back in the day would later grow to appreciate making healthier choices in how I eat or make fitness a priority in my lifestyle or learn to heal emotionally and all those kinds of positive things that keep us well—it was becoming clearer and clearer to me that my mindset *had* to change.

But finding that clarity can be like a jungle sometimes.

In countries where monkey populations are so huge that they're considered a local nuisance by the neighboring towns, trappers have learned to use the monkeys' psychology to trap them. They use sugar cubes as bait, allowing the monkeys easy access to the sugar through holes cut in gourds just big enough for their hands to squeeze in and grab it. It's not long before whole monkey tribes become addicted to the sweet bait. The hole is large enough for the monkey to get his hand inside, but not large enough for the monkey's fist to come back out while still holding on to the sugar cubes. So, the monkey gets caught by the trap, because he won't let go. The monkey wants that familiar treat more than he values his own safety and freedom.

Social conditioning kind of works like those traps, tempting us with sugar-coated, often false notions of the world around us and how it works. Being attached to what you are familiar with can be comforting and feel safe, but it can easily become a trap in itself. Through the lens of the game, or the socially constructed status quos, we see things how we are conditioned and trained to see them. We see the sweet we want but we don't realize the trap. We get stuck in the identities of our programming. We become attached to dysfunctional thought patterns and beliefs, and we end up trapped like a monkey does with his stubborn fist full of sugar cubes. Instead of using the power of our own intelligence to save ourselves and let go of potentially dangerous ideas and ideals, we suffer, and we miss out on alternative solutions and opportunities that could free us up in new ways. And by the way, it's interesting to note that human beings share roughly 99 percent of the exact same DNA as chimpanzees. There is only 1 percent genetic difference, yet there is, at least theoretically, a vast amount of difference between the intellectual sophistication of a human and of a chimpanzee. But sometimes it's harder to tell.

I was the epitome of that proverbial monkey, sleepwalking through life, holding on to a dysfunctional street-life mindset like a sugar cube. There were some valuable tests and takeaways I got from the streets, too, I ain't going to front, but where I was ultimately headed was not going to turn out well. Sometimes just letting go of what's not good for us is the best thing we can do for our lives in the long run. The trials and tribulations and tough times we go through are actually some of the best teachable moments. As we become more self-aware and start to shake off the shackles of our "environmentality"—the way we think and live based on the limiting conditions of our environment— we are able to consciously grow and take care of ourselves better. You don't have to just be the *product* of your environment; you can also be the *producer* of it.

Knowing the L.E.D.G.E.

You ain't got to be locked up to be in prison. We can be mentally incarcerated by the thoughts and the social conditioning that we allow to control us. During that "sit down" in the county for those months, I was able to put in perspective how the conditions of my environment were influencing my mindset and choices for the worse. And at the same time, I was becoming more and more aware of how I could use the power of my own mind to influence my conditions—for the better.

Until we learn otherwise, our mindsets are shaped by the world and how we perceive the conditions around us, and that mindset shapes our identity. And how we self-identify shapes our choices. In my youth, the street-life mentality was my framework, so I made choices from that limited knowledge of myself. Maybe you are in that same space right now or maybe your mindset is shaped by some other limiting view of your self-identity—it could be all sorts of conditioning that we take on as who we are without fully realizing it.

Mindset frames your worldview, and out of your worldview, you make your choices—and our choices ultimately shape our lives. Once we recognize this, the floodgates of possibilities open up. This is when we can really start to take ownership of our mindset in our lives to improve our well-being. Knowledge of self begins when we stop sleep-walking through life and we start to become more self-aware and conscious of our actions. We have to be willing to let go of what we think we already know. Let go of the limiting boxes. We have to be willing to admit when we are wrong. The more we really know and understand ourselves, the better choices we can make. The conditions and challenges we face definitely shape us, but I've seen that it's really the quality of our choices *in* the circumstances that matters most.

Deprogramming

So, I was still in jail, but I wasn't going crazy. I was waking up. I was just at the very beginning of a lifelong process but that time in jail was just the call to action I needed to start getting my mind right.

Many years later, I came across the work of author Vishen Lakhiani and his eye-opening concept of "culturescape," which he uses to define the world of race, class, nationality, ethnicity, religion, and business around us with its social conditioning, long-held beliefs, and limiting behaviors—the "bullshit rules," as he calls them. What we by default see as right and wrong, what's expected of us, how we are expected to think, how we define respect, how we dress, how we talk, how we feel we're supposed to react in different scenarios—these are our culturescapes, or what I call "boxes of behavior" that can limit our ability to make conscious choices that are in our best interest.

Lakhiani continues to break things down: By intentionally thinking and living outside of the expectations of this unconscious "programming," we start to wake up. Instead of being controlled by the identities of the world around us, we start to focus on an identity in the world that we consciously choose. The more we understand what has shaped and motivated us—for the good or for the bad—the better we can make wiser and healthier choices going forward.

Building Self-Awareness

No health goals are sustainable without the right mindset. Mindset and mental well-being are the foundation of all other aspects of health, 'cause if the mind ain't right, we won't have the awareness, the discipline, the balance, or the internal motivation to consistently make the choices that are in our best interest. Self-awareness creates the space and gives us the intel to decode and recode ourselves.

It starts with a reality check of where we are and gaining an understanding why we are the way we are, and then making a decision to learn better and do better, creating a vision of a healthier version of our lives that we can aspire to. We can remix our mindset, beliefs, and behaviors anytime we choose. It's really an empowering, revolutionary process.

At birth, my pops named me Clay after my granddad, but I changed it to Khnum as I gained more knowledge about my cultural roots as an African descendent. Khnum is the principle of creativity and building, symbolized by the ram-headed master potter in ancient Egyptian cosmology, who spun clay on his cosmic potter's wheel to mold the bodies and spirits of man come to life. We are all like this in the sense that we can shape and reshape our lives for the better. Unlearning, unpacking, and understanding what impacts and shapes us and how we in turn are impacting and shaping our own experiences is key. Through our mindsets, like master potters, the form our life takes on is in our own hands.

Living and learning produce self-knowledge that enables us to move forward from the limitations that no longer serve us. Life is a classroom. You can learn from any situation. Every experience is a part of the curriculum. The more we pay attention to our experiences and catch the jewels from them, the better we can understand their valuable lessons.

I call it *knowing the ledge*, with the acronym L.E.D.G.E.—for Learn Every Day Grow Evolve—and it's a lifelong pledge to keep learning every day, growing, and evolving.

It's about always remaining a student of life.

CHAPTER 2

White-Belt Mentality

Despite my firm convictions, I have always been a man who tries to face facts, and to accept the reality of life as new experience and new knowledge unfolds it. I have always kept an open mind, which is necessary to the flexibility that must go hand in hand with every form of intelligent search for truth.

—*Malcolm X*

When Malcolm X broke with the Nation of Islam in 1964, he had been a devoted member and leader of the movement for more than a decade. His impact had been so undeniable that he was known as one of the most influential members of the Nation, ranking just behind its founder, Elijah Muhammad. For twelve years, his voice, image, thoughts—everything about him—were synonymously linked with the NOI. Imagine then, how much personal integrity it took for Malcolm to take the stand he took when he ultimately left the Nation. Here was a proud Black man who, since the early 1950s, had led the charge as the organization's national spokesperson and helped build it into a powerful movement across the US, well-known and respected around the world. He was THE voice and face of the movement. It would have been so much easier, and less dangerous, for him to just be quiet about the upsetting personal things he learned about his leader and teacher Elijah Muhammad. He could have chosen to deny it or ignore what had come to light and kept it to himself. He didn't have to publicly acknowledge the radical change of perspective on race that his pilgrimage to Mecca had produced in him. But being the man of integrity that he was, Malcolm humbled himself to the truth as he saw it, and changed with change, just as he did when, as Detroit Red, he humbled himself in prison to become the minister Malcolm X, the same way he was willing to adopt a position of growth and change after coming back from Mecca as el-Hajj Malik el-Shabazz.

What Malcolm X possessed was the integrity and confidence to know when and how to become a student in life again and again. Thankfully, we don't all have to face the same level of consequences that Malcolm did for changing his mind, but when it comes to personal growth and healthy living, being able to humble ourselves and embrace a beginner's mind, or what I call a white-belt mentality, is powerful and necessary. Like 2Pac said, "even the genius asks questions."

I'm willing to bet you know what a black belt is even if you never studied martial arts a day in your life. A black belt is what all the students strive to be. It is the most popular symbol of expertise in martial arts. The black belt represents knowledge and skill. The white belt, on the other hand, represents the opposite. The white belt is the first belt someone starting a martial art practice will receive; it signifies the beginning of a new journey. In other words, the white belt is the beginner, the novice. In the martial-arts training space, or dojo, the white belt is the most unskilled and untrained. He's like an unformed lump of clay. But the good thing is you know that as a white belt in the dojo, you don't know. And when you know you don't know you are in the best frame of mind to be able to grow by listening and learning and asking questions. You're open to considering all kinds of possibilities. Ain't no room for the ego because the beginner is getting humbling reminders in class daily when confronted with greater skills and more advanced knowledge. Whatever you think you know is easily yielded when you're put on your ass, over and over and over. You're forced to swallow your pride when confronted with challenges that require greater skills than you actually have. A dude who's got a little bit of hands in the street and expects to dominate advanced students in the dojo will quickly realize that all the wild bravado in the world ain't got shit on properly executed techniques. As a white belt, you have no choice but to be humble, open, and receptive to learn. But dig this: one of the greatest philosophical insights that the martial arts teach is that *in every disadvantage there is an advantage.* So, the fact that the white-belt student is a beginner means that he or she has the most to learn—and that's why the white belt has the *greatest potential* in the dojo.

Beginner's Advantage

> Instead of establishing rigid rules and separative thoughts, we should look within ourselves to see where our particular problems lie and our cause of ignorance. You see, ultimately all type of knowledge simply means self-knowledge. You must look for truth yourself and directly experience every minute detail for yourself.
>
> —*Bruce Lee*

Maintaining a white-belt mentality in life and in your well-being practice gives you an advantage because you are honest with yourself about what is working and what's not working, and it's only from that space of awareness and realness that we can actually grow and develop. We have a tendency as humans to cling to the familiar way as

THE WAY. But in doing so, we can easily get stuck repeating patterns that may or may not actually be working out for us. We too often block our blessings by thinking we already know what's correct instead of being open and listening, living, and learning to receive insight that could greatly benefit our lives. How many traditions and cycles in our families and communities do we continue just because that's the way it's been done, even when we see it hasn't worked out so well? People say the older we get the more we get stuck in our ways but shit, it's plenty of young folks in their own way, too. You can benefit from a white-belt mentality at any and every age.

As the white belt, you are a fresh canvas. Nothing is decided. Everything is new. Anything is possible. Many people think that admitting that they have more to learn is a weakness, but owning our ignorance is actually one of the smartest things we can do. And when it comes to making healthy choices for your life, the humility to recognize and acknowledge that there's always more to know and room to grow is one of the greatest strengths you can have.

A white-belt mentality recognizes there is no one right way to accomplish anything. Everybody is unique and learns differently, truth is relative, things change, context matters—there's always more than one way up the mountain! There are conventional systems of knowledge and alternative systems of knowledge. You can learn from scientific methods, and you can also learn through your own spiritual instincts. You can learn through your own experiences and those of others. You can learn from instruction, and you can learn through intuition. You can consult an expert or an oracle or both. Just as there are a gang of ways of living, there are mad avenues for learning. As things change, people change, information changes, situations and circumstances change—our minds and behaviors can and should also change, adapt, and respond accordingly. Everything changes. The ability to either change or adapt to one's environment is actually a sign of intelligence and resilience, not weakness.

Many impactful people throughout time have acknowledged that humility is the beginning of wisdom. Mike Tyson said, "If you're not humble, life will visit humbleness upon you." Albert Einstein put it this way: "A true genius admits that he/she knows nothing." In her classic song "On and On," my homey Erykah Badu said, "The man that knows something knows that he knows nothing at all."

That's the white-belt mentality. It allows us to break out of ignorant patterns and cycles, acknowledge our own strengths and shortcomings, stay curious, and cultivate an open-minded perspective as a lifelong attitude. It's cool to respect the knowledge and expertise that the black belt represents, but it's about putting some perspective and respect on that white belt, too. After all, a black belt is just a white belt that has kept on learning.

Testing Our Theories

Even though I've been expressing my twin passions for hip-hop and healthy living for decades now, and there are people who think of me as a health and fitness expert—some even have gone so far as to say I'm a guru, which I never claim to be—I see myself as a student of life, sharing my notes with my fellow classmates. I'm always reevaluating ideas and considering multiple ways of doing things. I've come to see that acknowledging and exploring my own ignorance is a great source of inspiration and insight as I continue to learn and evolve.

One of the ways I continue to learn, grow, and evolve on the daily is through reading.

My mom taught me how to read early, at like two years old. She'd give me words to find and I'd make a game of pointing those words out in newspapers, magazines, and dictionaries. Even in my "fuck school" phase, or jail, I never lost my love for learning and reading. Today, I probably have amassed over three thousand books.

On tour, the homies nicknamed me Booker "G" Washington because I'd always travel with more books than clothes in my luggage.

I carry a book with me everywhere, like I used to carry my pistol. If I know I'mma be waiting in line at a bank, or in the carpool line while picking my son up from school, or doing any errand where I might have an opportunity to study, I'll definitely have a book within reach. And if I don't have a physical book on deck, I'll always have my earbuds handy to tap into an audiobook on my phone. I prefer physical books, but audiobooks are so convenient because you can listen and learn while your hands are busy. Reading is one of my favorite forms of entertainment as well as one of the most convenient ways I broaden my knowledge base.

But it ain't just about being book smart. We can memorize all kinds of facts and claim we have knowledge, but unless we test that theoretical knowledge in the context of the living, moving, nuanced, and changing circumstances of real life, it's just theory—and as Fred Hampton of the Black Panther Party so eloquently put it, "theory with no practice ain't shit." We have to continually put our theories to the test in real situations to test their validity. And what used to work yesterday might not work today or tomorrow.

These days, in the wellness space, there are all kinds of diets and workouts claiming to be the best thing ever. Everybody wants to prove their method is the right way or the only way. I say soak it up, be a sponge to it all—it's healthy to see many sides and be well-rounded. We don't need to be fanatics about any one perspective to the point where we get stuck in our own ignorance. There are many ancient wisdom traditions and other old-school ways of thinking and going about things that are tried and tested and remain valid in our lives from generation to generation, and it is a beautiful thing to honor, preserve, and implement the richness of our cultural legacies. Yet we should also respect the fact that for culture to remain relevant it must be updateable, upgradeable, and applicable for the changing modern world. Like software updates on our phones and computers, it's good to update our mental operating systems often. We want to use the best and wisest practices that we can, whether old or new. As Bruce Lee would say, and you'll hear me say this again and again: "Absorb what is useful, discard what is useless and add what is specifically your own."

So, if we can say as a metaphor the black belt represents the skills, knowledge, and answers we all seek for well-being in our lives, then learning to continually ask ourselves better and better questions is a great way for the white belt to make progress in that direction.

A Question of Power

I took a course in holistic life coaching some years back, and one of the most impactful takeaways I still use to this day is a tool called the "power question." Authors Jerold Panas and Andrew Sobel coined the term in their best-selling book by the same title. Power questions, put simply, are questions that are engaging, thought provoking, and open up empowering possibilities.

For example, let's take a common statement like, "I just don't like working out," and rephrase it as a power question. It might sound something like this: "What's something I can do to better enjoy working out?"

Power questions are designed to uncover and get to the root cause of important issues, decisions, problems, and dilemmas and inspire us to look past what is and see what can be possible through our own actions or a shift in perspective. Power questions reframe perspectives in proactive and transformative ways. The right question, a powerful question, can cascade into a wave of actionable insight and forward momentum in your life.

Powerless statements and questions, on the other hand, only have one answer that is readily available, so there's no inspiration to dig deeper. If I were to ask you a closed-ended question that just has a yes or no answer, that won't pull out any particularly useful insights or help you to imagine things differently. But power questions are like prompts designed to draw out new and more helpful ways of seeing things.

Practicing reframing our preconceived notions and limiting conclusions, thoughts, and self-talk into the form of power questions gives us the chance to expand our perspective and our options. The right question can help you reframe a scenario in a way that reveals a new solution you might not have seen otherwise. They offer us the opportunity to consider alternate endings to life's situations and circumstances.

Here are eight ways I strive to apply a white-belt mindset in my life, followed by power questions that correspond to each of the takeaways:

1. **REMOVE THE FILTER.** If you root your identity in fixed ideas, you will inevitably get stuck when those notions aren't flexible enough to align with reality effectively. When you feel stagnant, confused, frustrated, or things just seem unclear, there's a good chance your conditioned self-identity is getting in the way of you seeing what could be possible for you, without that filter limiting your options. Strive to identify which aspects of your conditioned "environmentality" are influencing your perspective. Investigate the cause of your own ignorance by asking yourself what you are not seeing because of your attachments to certain preferences.
   Power Questions: What cultural ideas and influences are shaping, framing, or even limiting my perspective and options in my current situation? How's that working out? Which things are helping? Are there other ideas beyond my cultural norms to consider that may be helpful, and, if so, what are they?

2. **HUMBLE UP.** Self-improvement begins with the humility to recognize that there is always room to grow. Acknowledging the limits of what we know in a given scenario frees our minds to learn and make power moves forward.

   Power Question: What could my own arrogance and assumptions be in the way of, or be blocking, right now?

3. **REEVALUATE.** What works in one scenario may not work in another; and what worked in the past may not continue to work in the future, and vice versa.

   Power Questions: What patterns am I repeating that are no longer serving me or the others around me? What actions have worked out well for me in similar scenarios?

4. **ARGUE THE OPPOSITE.** Be well-rounded. It's fine to have your notions, but the more perspectives you can appreciate, the better and more options you give yourself to flow with life.

   Power Questions: What if the opposite were true? What else am I not seeing or considering? Can more than one perspective be valid in this scenario?

5. **TRY A "YES, AND" PERSPECTIVE.** There's more than one way up the mountain. Respect and appreciate different ways of doing things.

   Power Question: What other ways might also work?

6. **THEORY—PRACTICE—THEORY.** Live, learn, adapt, and repeat. Trust your own experience, but also pick up game from the experiences of others and examples all around you.

   Power Questions: How can I test my belief or assumption? How is my current theory/belief/perspective working out in my life? What adjustments can I make to something I hold true that might help achieve different results?

7. **TAKE CLASSES.** Learn new skills; budget time, energy, and money for continuing your education. It doesn't have to be formal institutional education, it can be in any form—online, or even from a friend. One of my favorite ways to learn is to hire consultants. You pay for an hour of their time, ask questions, and take notes.

    Power Questions: How could I increase my knowledge or skills in this area? How would improving or developing more skills in a particular area be of benefit? Who could I consult on this issue that has expertise I don't? What key words can I google to get more insight on a given issue or interest? What kind of classes online or in person are available so I can continue my education in a particular direction? Who do I know that can teach me or give me insight on a particular question I may have?

8. **PUT IT TO THE TEST.** Always be willing to reevaluate and reconsider your perspectives and options, because things can change, nuances matter, and real-life wisdom is not fixed—it's fluid.

    Power Questions: How can I test my assumptions? What have I learned from my tests and experience? What adjustments will be helpful?

CHAPTER 3

Right Mind: Building Mental & Emotional Fitness

Emancipate yourselves from mental slavery; none but ourselves can free our minds.

—*Bob Marley*

This may be a controversial statement, and I hope you'll receive it in the constructive sense and context that I mean it: The greatest slavery in the history of the world, that human beings still suffer the tyranny of every day, was not chattel slavery, or economic slavery, or even sexual slavery—though all those still contribute to what I'm about to say. I believe the most oppressive system of slavery the world has ever seen is the state of believing in the illusion of control that stress has over our lives. When we give our power over to stress, it becomes the ultimate oppressive force and monster in our own minds, and it's one of the toughest obstacles we will ever face.

You might not immediately agree, but I feel like we instinctively know this; but at the same time, we feel like everybody else reacts this way, so it's normalized and many of us feel that it's unrealistic to think things could be different. "If you're human, that's just the way it is," we tell ourselves to rationalize the control stress has over our lives. And so, we're stuck in our different degrees of emotional suffering largely because we don't or won't take the time, or don't have the know-how, to break the cycle. But because of the epidemic-size devastation and havoc stress wreaks in our lives, in our relationships, and on our mental, emotional, and physical well-being, stress is an opponent worthy of much study and much respect.

In his book *Stress Free for Life*, Ra Un Nefer Amen suggests stress is the leading contributor to all sorts of preventable chronic and acute illnesses, mental disorders, and even lowered IQ. He proposes that stress can and must be prevented and eliminated, not just managed. He explains the reason that we struggle to do so is because we misunderstand what stress actually is. We might know when we are feeling "stressed," but do we know what stress actually consists of?

Stress is a combination of thoughts, emotions, and bodily responses. One of the things renowned scientist Ivan Pavlov demonstrated with his experiments in the 1890s—in which he noticed that, after some conditioning, dogs would salivate at the sound of a ringing bell—was that our thoughts, emotions, and bodily responses are *connected*. In 1935, Harvard psychologist Walter B. Cannon described stress as a disturbing force that upsets a person's usual balance or homeostasis, a term he coined for the general sense of ease and flow of our internal functions—temperature, blood pressure, pH balance of the blood, pulse, and so forth. However, thousands of years before this, Chinese physicians had already used the term *tai chi* to describe this state of inner balance, and they taught that stress was its chief disturbance.

In Western society, we have been conditioned to believe that stress is caused by stressful things outside our control that "stress us," but let's question that for a sec. If stress is actually *caused* by outside factors, then why is it that people get stressed by a particular challenging situation while others don't? That means that, as hard as it might be to accept for some of us, the truth is that situations don't automatically cause stress; it is our own response to the situation that causes it.

However, there's a positive aspect: if our responses to situations cause stress, our responses can also prevent stress. Stress is not a thing in and of itself, caused by outside "stressors" (a stressful relationship, a stressful job, stressful financial times, or a stressful day). Stress is a mental, emotional, and physical reaction to those situations and circumstances, which we cause or prevent by how we perceive, process, and respond to them. That doesn't mean that certain situations are not challenging or difficult, but there is a difference between responding to challenging situations in a stressed-out way and responding from a stable space of peace within ourselves—a big difference. You've probably heard the idea that in "stressful" situations we have only a few choices: either fight or flight. In more modern circles, they've added "freeze"—where you get so overwhelmed that you don't respond either way, like a deer in headlights—and "fawn"—where you try to appease whomever or whatever is causing you the stress. So, within the parameters of these limited reactions, we can only go to battle against whatever we are feeling; try to suppress, run away, and avoid it; do nothing at all; or be appeasing.

But there's another option—we can flow.

A BETTER STRESS RESPONSE

Lack of knowledge, skill, or understanding; malnutrition; too little or too much movement; lack of rest; lack of inspiration; doing too much or not doing what we need to do are all contributing factors and triggers to the stress we experience in our lives. But we are not powerless to fix that. Responding with flow instead of stress is an attainable skill through practice.

In my own experiences, I've come to realize that stress is one of my best teachers. When I'm triggered by life events and I start to feel that disturbance of my peace, those triggers that I used to call stresses and stressors, I now see them as reminders to return to my practice of flow and choose to respond mindfully instead of losing my shit and spazzing out. At least, most of the time.

We experience mental and emotional stress when we don't have the willingness or the skills to let go of what's not serving us and reframe things in constructive, resilient ways. Learning effective techniques to prevent and transcend the stress that our unskillful reactions create in our lives is a major key—to borrow a phrase from DJ Khaled. I've found that embodying the posture of the white belt and posing power questions is super helpful for my mental health.

The Body Keeps the Score

Managing our own emotions and responding skillfully to the emotions of others is key in maintaining a healthy mindset. Stress provides the perfect opportunity to challenge and strengthen our mental fitness. In fact, how well we manage our response to the so-called stressors in our lives is a good indicator of the level of our mental and emotional fitness.

Now raise your hand if you struggle with that. My hand is up, too. It's something everyone battles to different degrees. When I'm good, I'm great. I'm in my right mind and I'm flowing and glowing. But when I'm stressed, I feel horrible. It's like there is a hot, irritating field of negative resistance that's weighing my mind and spirit down. I can feel heat in my back and sometimes it shows up as aches or tension in my head or chest. It's like a terrible storm that clouds my mind with frustration and discontent. I don't sleep as well, it's harder to focus, I lose my inner peace, and my mood turns to shit. I'm not in my right mind. And that cycle of feeling great then horrible wears and tears on you. After living in that back and forth, up-and-down cycle over and over, you want a release from that cycle. You want to get off that ride and find a more stable and peaceful way to live. That's why I've learned to appreciate being proactive with my mental health so much.

Our bodies respond to the way we think, feel, and act. That's what is known as the mind-body connection. When we don't feel good emotionally or mentally, our physical health suffers, too. We're more susceptible to getting colds and other infections during emotionally difficult times. When we're feeling stressed, anxious, or upset, we may not feel like exercising, eating nutritious foods, or taking care of ourselves in the best ways. We often reach for alcohol, tobacco, and other drugs to try and "take the edge off life," but you already know those substances are double-edged swords with all sorts of negative side effects.

But in our right minds—when we are fully present, mindful, and not controlled by stressful emotions—we can better weather the storms of life. Another reason that mindset matters to our state of physical health and well-being is because our thoughts and emotions are not only *psychological*; they are also *physiological*. Thoughts and emotions have corresponding biochemical effects on our physical states, meaning how we think and feel physically affects us. Our mental and emotional states correspond and influence our physical states and vice versa. It's all interconnected.

Sangfroid

Snoop Dogg once shared a story: A cofounder of the Crips, Stanley Tookie Williams, was on death row in California. Days before he was executed, Snoop went in to visit the OG and lend his support to the campaign to save his life, and they had a powerful convo. Snoop was so impressed by Tookie's composure in the situation that he had to ask him how he could be so cool and collected, facing death by execution in a matter of days. Tookie explained to Snoop that he practiced *sangfroid*, a French term that pretty much means "calm under pressure." Tookie said he taught himself that skill over time so that whatever he must face—even death—he could do so with acceptance, grace, and dignity. That story has stuck with me.

We don't have to control our every emotion, and it's not about fighting or fleeing away from what we feel, but we can learn how to continue our flow regardless of our circumstances. Flowing is about first acknowledging how we feel and allowing ourselves to accept how we feel, and then mindfully choosing how to respond to those feelings in a way that's in the best interest of the situation and our inner well-being. We don't have to take on the reactionary identity of what we are feeling. Instead of "I AM ANGRY," we can reframe it and say, "I feel anger right now." This subtle shift in perspective puts the power to choose our response back in our hands instead of being enslaved by automatic emotional (stressful) reactions. Feelings come and go if we let them. We are not our feelings; they happen within the atmosphere of our awareness but we are the perceiver of the feelings, not the embodiment of the feelings. Our true self remains while feelings come and go. It's as if we are the sky and the feelings are the weather. We can remain above the clouds.

That don't mean it's fun to live through a hurricane. Of course it's easier to live life when the sun is shining and the weather is clear, to quote another Bob Marley lyric. Is it easier to live life when I'm happy compared to when I feel stressed? Fasho. But if we let our emotional weather determine our days and decisions or dictate what we can and cannot get done, we suffer for lack of self-control. My mom always reminds me when I'm in a funk that "this too shall pass." She'd always say, "If you're going through hell, keep going." It's been said for good reasons that emotions are great servants but poor masters. Emotions aren't bad, they are powerful—and with great power comes great responsibility. With practice, I've seen that negative feelings don't automatically dictate and dominate my mood all the time. Dr. Richard J. Davidson, a neuroscientist at the University of Wisconsin–Madison, stated that his research points to the importance of mind training in changing brain circuits in a way that will promote positive responses. If you practice, you can actually get better at it. His research has found a link between upbeat mental states and improved health, including lower blood pressure, better blood sugar levels, reduced risk for heart disease, and longer life.

Maintaining Your Right Mind

> Positive psychology is a scientific approach to studying human thoughts, feelings, and behavior, with a focus on strengths instead of weaknesses, building the good in life instead of repairing the bad, and taking the lives of average people up to "great" instead of focusing solely on moving those who are struggling up to "normal."
>
> —*Courtney E. Ackerman, paraphrasing*
> *Christopher Peterson*

There are so many insights from neuroscience and psychology that are useful for everyday life. The field of positive psychology, founded by Dr. Martin Seligman, is a distinct branch of psychology that focuses on human strengths and virtues, and what makes us happy, resilient, exceptional, and function at our best, unlike conventional psychology, which generally focuses on mental illness, trauma, suffering, and things that malfunction in the human mind.

In short, positive psychology emphasizes what I've been getting at all along in this chapter: building mental and emotional fitness—what I like to call right mind. I've learned to check my own mental fitness on a regular basis by assessing my mind in four key areas: strength, flexibility, endurance, and vitality. Self-reflective check-ins are key to my mental-health regimen.

Mental Strength. This means clarity, resilience, discipline, and follow-through. That's my zone state. When I can concentrate and focus well, I can handle the heavy lifting of life positively with a sense of purpose and meaning.

Mental Flexibility. I gauge this by how well I'm flowing with life, how optimistic, adaptive, and graceful I am during challenges, how open I'm able to be to perspectives other than my own, and how creative and experimental I'm willing to be in a given situation that requires it.

Mental Endurance. I can tell I'm in good shape in that area when I don't give up easily in the face of adversity. I keep my head in the game, and I'm able to stay true to my commitments in the face of trials and tribulations, challenges and changes with resilience and perseverance.

Mental Vitality. This encompasses an overall feeling of peace of mind, the natural result of an ability to free up more of my mental and emotional bandwidth by giving my mind rest and relaxation from stress. When I'm in that state of inner vitality, I can exercise my intuition, insight, and gratitude at a high level. I'm more empathic, and I feel more compassion and love.

That's what being in my right mind feels and looks like for me. But I don't have to tell you that sometimes life can hit hard and get the best of us and we can get knocked off-balance. I know I'm mentally and emotionally out of shape when self-doubt is kicking my ass, it's hard to focus, my discipline slips, and I'm not able to concentrate on what matters. I know I'm mentally and emotionally out of shape when I feel stuck and stagnant, when my stubbornness or rigid point of view is getting in the way, when I feel out of flow, and when I'm frustrated and in disharmony with what's going on in my life. I recognize I'm mentally and emotionally out of shape when I'm short on patience, short-tempered, and shortsighted, when I can't appreciate the big picture because I'm too distracted by short-term circumstances. I know I'm mentally and emotionally out of shape when I'm becoming pessimistic, expecting the worst, assuming the negative, and overreacting immaturely to challenges instead of mindfully responding.

If you are like me, it's always a work in progress. And just like the only way the body stays fit and in shape is if we consistently work out, it's the same for the mind. We have to consistently train the mind right, to sustain the balance and the benefits of being in our right minds.

And this is where the practice of mindfulness fits into mental and emotional fitness.

Mindfulness

> The positive net-result of mindfulness might be that the people you engage feel non-threatened, accepted, heard, and relaxed upon interacting with you. Meanwhile, you would most likely be unaffected by interactions with others, remaining fully aware of yourself throughout each experience.
>
> —*Paul Wagner*

Mindfulness is paying real attention to our lives in the moments that we live them. It's knowing the difference between when we are present and responding deliberately and when we are distracted and reacting unskillfully. How many times have you said to yourself,

"If I had been in my right mind, I wouldn't have done this or that"? Or, "Had I been in my right mind, I could've done something differently"? Mindfulness is a skillful way of making more of an effort to catch those moments in the moment instead of after the fact. When we're mindful, we can observe how certain states of mind even arise in the first place.

There's no quick-fix magic formula for practicing mindfulness—that I know of, at least—you just have to practice staying in observation mode of your own thoughts, feelings, and actions. Emotional stress and drama can seem like weeds in your life garden that just keep growing. Mindfulness is tending to your inner garden so that the seeds you want to flourish are nourished and the weeds that need to be uprooted are removed on a regular basis. The more mindful we are, the less regrets we have in life and the better we're able to navigate and make choices that reflect our best intentions and best interests—in the moment, instead of in hindsight.

I'm not a Buddhist, but I might consider myself "Buddh-*ish*." In Buddhism, Right Mindfulness is one of the essential tenets of the Buddha's Noble Eightfold Path. Living life in a state of mindfulness promotes relaxation, awareness, efficiency, and control.

Right mind combines both intellectual and emotional intelligence. Emotional intelligence is the set of skills that allow you to understand, use, and manage your own emotions in constructive ways to release, relieve, or prevent stress; communicate effectively; recognize and empathize with other people's emotions; navigate and overcome challenging circumstances; and prevent, defuse, or resolve unnecessary conflicts and drama.

Let's unpack some tools from the mental gym bag. Here are eleven practical ways to assist our right-mind practice.

1. **TRUST THE LAW OF AFFIRMATION.** Affirmations are statements phrased in the present tense that train your mind

to operate from a positive, empowered attitude and perspective. Breathe slowly and deeply to establish a calm, receptive frame of mind, followed by relentless repetition of the phrase until it becomes tattooed into your "mental muscle memory." The law of repetition establishes momentum, atmosphere, and resonance. When you repeat your affirmation, it leaves a resonance of that intention in your subconscious mind. With enough repetition, you start to subconsciously operate from the influence of your affirmation. It's like you are manually writing code for yourself. Our thoughts are powerful, and the ones we repeat the most will flourish in our lives. Negative thoughts can't thrive in a positively reinforced mind. Affirm and repeat what you want to speak into life.

2. **CHANT YOUR MANTRAS.** Similar to affirmations, mantras like the ancient sacred word *om*, and many others, also use the law of repetition. But instead of using words or phrases, mantras are sounds that are repeated to kind of sweep the mind and purify your inner space with their sound vibration. Think of a mantra like a metronome; you can bob your head along with it to get yourself in a certain zone or frame of mind. Chanting these sounds is a powerful way to sweep out your mind and reset your vibes when you need it.

3. **GRATITUDE ATTITUDE.** Practicing gratitude daily is a great way to shift your focus onto appreciating the lotus of life instead of wallowing in the mud. Giving thanks before meals is one way I stay consistent daily with expressing gratitude for what I'm thankful for. Another good practice for when you are feeling off-balance is to keep a gratitude journal. Make a list of things you are grateful for. You can even keep these lists on your phone. When you get in a rut, review these lists— they come in handy reminding us how blessed we truly are and to stay focused on what truly matters.

4. **SWEAT THE TECHNIQUE.** Sweating is definitely a go-to I use as an outlet during highly challenging times. I can't tell you how many times an argument has fueled an epic gym session or inspired a beautiful long-distance run to release tension in a constructive manner. Physical exercise also helps me overcome anxiety. I always like to pump out a gang of push-ups before performances or important meetings. When we sweat, we release not only physical toxins but toxic states of mind as well. Hot yoga classes, sweat-lodge ceremonies, some impromptu calisthenics, or regular visits to the steam room are great ways to use sweat to support your mental fitness.

5. **CIRCLE UP WITH FAMILY OR FRIENDS.** Building with the homies is a great way to take care of your mental health. Women often have "sister circles" where they confide in and support one another and celebrate their womanhood together. A lot of guys struggle with having folks they feel they can confide in, but I've learned it's crucial to have that support network in my life. Make an effort to get together with those you trust and chop it up in a heart-to-heart way. It's helpful and necessary for mental well-being. Holla at the homies.

6. **PRAYER IS POWERFUL.** Whatever your religious beliefs may be, there is something to be respected about prayer when it comes to practices that benefit your mind. Prayer involves an attitude of surrender, release, humility, and openness. By all means, if prayer is something that resonates with you, use it as a way of comforting your mind and relieving your concerns, and for spiritual connection with your understanding of source energy. When I first started flying a lot on airplanes, I noticed anxiety around the fear of plane crashes. But once I remembered my mama always taught me, *If you gonna pray don't worry and if you gonna worry don't pray,* it helped me relax into the fact that some things are out of our control. I'd

pray for safety and let it go. These kinds of prayers helped settle my mind.

7. **ROUTINES.** Life and all of its challenges can be chaotic at times and throw us off-balance. Having constructive routines in place provides a sense of stability, order, and familiarity amidst the chaos. Waking up, giving thanks, going for a jog, and doing my affirmations before breakfast is one of my routines that keeps me grounded, focused, and uplifted at the start of my day and sets a positive momentum for how I approach whatever the day brings.

8. **CHANGE YOUR ROUTINE.** Just as it's important to use routines to establish regularity and stability, it's also important to mix up your routines from time to time to avoid burnout, boredom, or plateaus. If you are usually a night owl, try waking up earlier. If you usually lift, try yoga. If you usually jog around your neighborhood, try different locations. Change can inspire you in ways you least expect.

9. **CLEAR THE CLUTTER.** Cleaning, clearing, and decluttering our spaces soothes something deep inside us. You probably already know how coming home to a messy kitchen or walking into a messy work space can dampen your mood, drain your energy, and aggravate and irritate your mind. Minimalists are one step ahead of the rest because they don't let stuff get in the way of their peace and happiness. Take a page from the minimalist mindset. When we clean up and clear out our physical and mental spaces, we let go and lighten up—and life opens up.

10. **GUIDED VISUALIZATION.** Guided visualizations are audio recordings that lead your imagination along on an inner experience with visual and sensual suggestions. When I want to channel a certain frequency of mind, I'll sometimes search YouTube for good guided visualizations. There are so many categories to choose from—success state of mind, confidence,

forgiveness, and creativity, just to name a few. The key is taking time to sift through them and choosing some good ones that resonate with you. I share some links to some that I like at the end of the book.

11. **PROFESSIONAL SUPPORT.** Even the GOATs have coaches. Life coaches and therapists are a great investment in your mental fitness game. They can help you learn tools to better understand and manage your emotions, how to be more effective in your work and life balance, and offer valuable feedback that you can't always do for yourself. You don't have to feel like something is off to get professional help. If you can swing it, having a life coach or therapist when things are going well only enhances your mental health.

CRUSH, KILL, DESTROY STRESS TOOL KIT

Make a list of things that help you stay zen'd up and keep stress away. You'll have a toolbox to refer to whenever you feel you need it.

Here's my personal list:

Rain sounds	Sex	Tai chi
Zazen	Herbs	Call a loved one
Shower	Calisthenics	Archery
Run	Read	Scooter ride
Drink water	Draw	Gym
Walk	Soup	Be in or near water
Sleep	Steam room	Listen to relaxing or
Hot tea	Tapping	inspiring music
Comedy	Watch boxing	
Hug	Go outside	

Mind Over Matter/s

We each have untapped mental powers that science is only beginning to understand and reveal, but what we know for sure is that mindset matters in every aspect of our health and well-being. Mental and emotional fitness is really the aim of a consistent mindfulness practice. Being more present to what's happening in the moment allows us to keep emotions in check, leave the past in the past, release anxieties about the future, stop the incessant inner criticism and self-judgment, refrain from judging others, and be better at responding wisely and deliberately instead of overreacting to life. If the mind is like a mirror reflecting our perceptions, then our Right Mindfulness practices polish the mind's mirror so we can see everything more clearly. Be clear on this: good health begins in the mind, and skillfully managing our mental and emotional energies and powers is one of the most important influences we can have on our overall well-being. Right mindset matters, as a result—we feel better, think better, sleep better, heal better, and live better. Even if it's just a teaspoon of better—and I'll break down what I mean by that in the next chapter—it can make a world of difference.

CHAPTER 4

How to Meditate:
A Teaspoon of Better

Meditation has been around since the beginning of recorded history, and probably long before that. It has a long-documented history of use in Africa, India, Asia, and the Americas. Today, it's more popular and scientifically supported than ever.

Originally, meditation was practiced to help deepen understanding of the sacred and mystical forces of life and fully awaken our self-actualization. Today, meditation is a complementary, mind-body medicine practice for increasing calmness and physical relaxation, improving psychological and emotional balance, coping with illness and stress, and enhancing overall health and well-being.

There are many myths floating around about meditation that make it more mysterious and confusing than it needs to be. I think many folks are confused about what it actually is, and still more folks feel like they've tried it but it hasn't worked for them. People falsely think meditation is about stopping the mind from thinking. Good luck with that! Contrary to popular myth, meditation isn't so much about *clearing* the mind as it is about experiencing *clarity* of mind.

THE NORTH STAR

George Mumford, author of *The Mindful Athlete*, the man who taught Kobe Bryant and Michael Jordan meditation, has said: "The hardest thing, after all the work and all the time spent on training and technique, is just being fully present in the moment. When things get tough and our bodies start to react, we need mindfulness to reset our internal north star. We need to be quiet, listen, and practice conscious breathing to bring ourselves back to the present moment and activate the parasympathetic nervous system, putting the brake on and slowing things down in our bodies."

An Introduction

The first time I heard of meditation is kind of fuzzy in my memory, but I'm pretty sure it was around the time I worked as a clerk at Amen-Ra's Bookshop in my senior year of high school. The owners, Drs. Dana and Shannon Dennard, were a married couple who were both clinical psychologists and Black Psychology professors at Florida A&M University. "Baba" Dennard, as I called him, mentored me at a really emotionally challenging period of my life.

I was dealing with a lot of pain, my brother was suffering drug addiction, and my parents had divorced. I'd been kicked out of Wakulla High School for reciting a rap at our first assembly observance of Black History Month, and so I had to catch a ride with a neighbor every morning to get dropped off to Rickards High, which was thirty miles away from where I lived. I was angry and frustrated with the systemic oppression that was becoming more and more clear to me every day. Getting active in the streets was my outlet for that angst and bottled-up aggression I felt.

My mom hooked a session up for me to chat with Dr. Dennard, at first as a therapist. She thought that speaking with a Black psychologist might be therapeutic and help me find ways to manage the constant rage and frustration I was dealing with at that time. Our sessions were surprisingly relaxed and light. He told me the rage I was feeling as a young Black male was understandable and he made me feel heard and supported. I felt like he saw potential in me that I couldn't fully see at the time in myself. Shit, he even offered me a job after our sessions ended and that's how I started working at Amen-Ra's. Baba Dennard was a yogi and a bit of a mystic, too. I honestly can't remember if he taught me to meditate specifically, but he was definitely one of the first people I knew and respected personally who even talked about meditation as a self-care practice. In jail I had those certain moments of transcendental focus that just kind of spontaneously happened. But it wasn't until years later that I slowly became more and more intentional about practicing meditation on a regular basis. I watched a martial arts documentary on Bruce Lee and they mentioned the word *zen*, and I was instantly drawn to it. I took that as a spark and went down the rabbit hole and read a gang of books on meditation to try and understand it intellectually. I wanted to separate the hocus-pocus stuff from the real-deal-Holyfield to get my own practical experience and see what kind of noticeable effects a consistent practice, if any, would have in my life. I took classes here and there around the city in New York. I went to lectures. Afya and I visited the Open Center in Manhattan to learn different approaches in the introductory courses they offered. I studied teachings from everyone from Sri Chinmoy to Deepak Chopra to Sadhguru to Ra Un Nefer Amen to Russell Simmons to George Mumford. I wasn't so much seeking or expecting any kind of grand enlightenment to come out of it as I was looking for a way to better manage my mind, access and explore more of my mental abilities, and experience less suffering from stress.

As I would sit to practice, I went through all the normal things that you go through when you start a meditation practice. You struggle with feeling like you're not doing it right. You get uncomfortable sitting; your feet and ankles and legs hurt and go to sleep on you. Your back aches. Your mind wanders like a toddler on the loose. I even wondered more than a few times if meditation wasn't anything more than a "think positive" hustle. Little by little though, as life kept happening and I found myself needing a way to try to relax and clear my head, I'd pick it back up.

And one day I had a kind of breakthrough.

I was in my bedroom sitting on the floor on my red meditation cushion, with no goal in mind, nothing I was trying to do or experience. I just felt called to the cushion. I was just sitting, noticing my breath coming in and out, and relaxing into that rhythm.

Then after a while there was this profound sense of peace.

I was alert and aware, but still totally relaxed. It felt like an indescribable relief and release, as if I was floating inside. I enjoyed that deeply serene and peaceful moment for however long it lasted and then naturally and gently came back into my "usual" state of consciousness. There were no great revelations, magical colors, or any other fantastical events in those beautiful moments, but something fundamental in my mindset had shifted. Being in that state I knew that inner peace is not only possible, but it's also very natural and awesome! It was as if right then somehow my mind's default setting was turned from a lean toward pessimism to a lean toward optimism. I don't know why, but I felt happy. For no particular reason. Just happy inside. I also had the realization in that experience that meditation was not something I needed to "try hard at" to reach a goal. It became clear to me that each meditation experience, whatever it may be, is the goal in itself. Every meditative experience is different, and the goal isn't to make a particular feeling happen every time, necessarily. The goal is to simply show up, sit, and be present for whatever the experience reveals. My practice became so much more meaningful to me when I released the anxiety around doing it right and accepted that the path *is* the practice. I didn't have to try to do anything except let it happen. I started to look forward to my daily practice and meditation has been a part of my lifestyle for many years now.

THE MEDITATION STATE

We have three general states of consciousness—awake, asleep, and meditation. One of the modes of energy that our brains run on is electricity, just as our smartphones, radios, TVs, and our other gadgets do. Electrical activity is measured in cyclic units of activity called hertz (Hz). The brain produces the awake state at an electrical output of at least thirteen Hz. To induce the sleep state, the electrical output of the brain must be between four and seven Hz or less—but not zero, or we'd be brain-dead. The meditation state is that range of electrical brain activity around anywhere from three to twelve Hz. Meditation is the sweet spot (and the procedure that trains the brain to enter it) of being in a deeply relaxed awakened state while at the same time not falling asleep. So, we get some of the regenerative and restorative effects of sleep while being alert and conscious and able to deeply focus at the same time.

Tapping In

> Take a pail of muddy water, sit it still for long enough, the mud will sink to the bottom on its own, and the water will become clearer by itself.
>
> —*A quote from a teaching at*
> *Dharma Jewel Monastery*

Breathing in intentional ways is at the core of meditation practices because of the breath-mind-body-connection. There's a traditional saying in some yoga practices that "as the breath goes, so does the mind." Deep, slow, and rhythmic breathing slows down our brain waves, triggers deep relaxation in our bodies, and quiets the emotional reaction–centers in our brains.

We actually meditate naturally and spontaneously several times throughout the day. Whenever we are completely engaged in a thought, or a television show, or any activity we are doing to the point where we lose awareness of ourselves and all else that is going on around us, we are meditating. All those external events, sounds, distractions, thoughts, and internal mental chatter that would usually be carrying our attention, is not a distraction in those times. Why? Because we're only paying attention to whatever has our complete focus. That's meditating. Human beings are natural meditators; we drift into it almost automatically under certain conditions. We only notice when we are coming out of the state (like if a commercial comes on, or we get distracted by a thought, etc.). It's interesting that we don't notice when we are going into the state as much. That's why advertisers take advantage of the unconscious attention we give to our favorite TV shows and social media feeds, and they hope to slip in their suggestive messaging while our conscious guard is down. But that's a whole other rabbit hole.

The point here is to say that we enter the meditation state several times a day automatically, and we can learn to enter it at will through various meditation techniques.

Getting into Practice

There are countless studies that prove how effective meditation is for lowering blood pressure, creating better sleep patterns, reducing stress, increasing focus, cultivating compassion, and more, but the biggest benefit for me has been just being more at peace and resilient in my everyday life and able to tap into my creativity pretty much at will.

I experiment with different approaches to meditation—mantras, guided, with music, without music. Over time I've been able to settle into my breathing and enter a kind of fertile, suggestive state, explore certain thoughts and feelings or creative ideas, and I've learned to use mantras and visualizations to seed my subconscious with what I want to manifest.

Emotionally, I have more awareness and self-control. Having a simple practice that I can always go to, that helps me re-center when I'm off-balance, that helps me find clarity when I'm confused, that helps me find peace when I'm stressed, has been a game changer for my growth.

I've taken meditation classes at monasteries like Dharma Jewel in Atlanta. Each class is led by female monks and lasts two hours. The first hour is dedicated to guided breath counting meditation practice, and the other hour is for a lecture on Buddhist principles and teachings like the Four Noble Truths, the Five Precepts, and the Eightfold Path.

I also attended meditation lectures at Emory University, including a powerful talk that was given by the Dalai Lama on the connections between scientific research and meditation. My good friend Classic Tone is a formal Zen student and has encouraged me with lots of Zen teachings and other gems and jewels for my practice. My meditation practice inspired Afya to find her own meditation practice and she loves to follow along to Deepak Chopra and Oprah's guided meditation series. We did those often as a family when our oldest son was growing up. At first, he would fall asleep in his meditation chair, but he has grown up to really value having those practices in his life, and now, in his twenties, he tells us often how much he appreciates our family's healthy traditions.

The Zazen Tradition

Of all the meditation practices I've experimented with, Zazen is one of the approaches that has stuck with me the most. My good friend Enensa sent me a twenty-minute track labeled "Zazen" that has a recording produced by his father (spiritual teacher and founder of the Ausar Auset Society, Ra Un Nefer Amen) that guides you through a controlled breathing practice with these binaural electronic pulses and bleeps in the background.

Binaural sounds allow us to take advantage of an illusion effect created by the brain when we listen to two tones with slightly different frequencies at the same time. Our brains interpret the two tones as a new frequency of its own. This new frequency is equal to the difference in hertz between the two original tones. When we listen to the sounds, our brain-wave activity adapts to match the frequency through the universal principle of entrainment, or the frequency-following effect. And that's why binaural tones help our minds enter certain mental states.

The Zazen method I practice uses binaural sounds coupled with a guided breathing pattern to lead you into a receptive state of mind. Once there, after about fifteen minutes or so, it prompts you to take advantage of being in that super suggestive state by visualizing yourself successfully overcoming emotional challenges you may be facing. It's like opening up a direct line of access to the subconscious mind and manually entering new code to consciously rewire your own behavior in a desired manner. I've probably done that particular meditation hundreds and hundreds of times, and it's the approach I've been most consistent with out of all the meditation methods I've experimented with. It's a big benefit to my life—it helps me better manage my emotions and keeps me in a positive, proactive mindset.

Make It Work for You

Your approach to meditation and what might work best for you is particular to you. Formal meditation classes are a great way to get acquainted with your own simple and relaxing practice. Many of the martial arts systems and yoga classes I've attended over the years have had some form of meditation incorporated. You have to explore different methods and techniques to find the ways that resonate best for you. You can use meditation to support all sorts of mental health attributes—confidence, self-love, self-awareness, happiness, peace, tranquility, and more—and there are all sorts of tried and tested methods to experiment with that can be helpful. I'm not a trained meditation teacher (yet!), but in my own personal experience, I do know there are some key fundamentals across the board that can be helpful to get you started.

A Teaspoon of Better

I worked with Toyota's Green Initiative as a healthy lifestyle–brand ambassador for a number of years. We were doing sustainability-themed social activations at large events like college basketball playoffs and big music festivals like Broccoli City Festival and Afropunk, and one of the dopest things about those experiences for me was that I got to put a lot of people on to meditation; for many of them, it was their first time ever practicing. For the initiative, I developed a super simple six-step introduction to meditation that I call "A Teaspoon of Better."

The name teaspoon of better comes from the initials T-S-P (teaspoon) and B-T-R (better), which represent each of the six aspects of a basic meditation practice. You can follow these six simple steps to begin exploring your own meditation practice:

1. **TIMER.** Set it and forget it. Set a timer for the desired amount of time you intend to practice, rather than letting yourself get distracted watching the clock. Begin with five minutes, and if that's too much, try sitting in silence for 60 seconds then build from there over time. Anywhere from five to twenty minutes is great for beginners.

2. **SPACE.** Find a comfortable space on the floor or in a chair, or even in the car. The main idea is to choose a comfortable space where you won't be interrupted. I know more than a few folks with kids who will squeeze in a few precious minutes of a meditation practice behind a locked bathroom door!

3. **POSTURE.** Sit with your palms faceup or facedown, either resting in your lap or on your thighs. Keep your back straight

and your shoulders relaxed to shake off any tension you might be holding in your upper body and to help steady your breathing. You can also use a wall to support your back—it's important to sit up straight in a royal position.

4. **BREATHING.** Breathe in and out through the nostrils. Breathe slowly and fully, deep down into the belly area. Your belly should rise when you inhale and flatten when you exhale. No need to force it! Stay relaxed, with attention present on your continuing breaths.

5. **THOUGHTS.** But what about all the nonstop thoughts and mental chatter? That's perfectly normal. As thoughts arise, the key is to notice them without becoming too engaged with them. If you get distracted away from your breath by thoughts or sounds around you or any other distraction, just gently return your focus back to your breath.

6. **REPS.** Every time you notice your attention has wandered away from the breath and you gently return your attention back to the breath, think of that like one repetition. Getting distracted doesn't mean you are doing it wrong. The distraction is actually an essential part of the practice, because noticing and returning back to the focus on your breath is the aim of the game. Repeat until the timer goes off.

Remember, there are many methods of meditation to explore. A teaspoon of better is just an intro, an easy way to remember the basics. It is a reminder to not worry so much about doing it "right." You will get distracted—that's a part of training your focus. It may seem impossible, but perfection ain't even the goal. It's the consistent stillness that brings the results.

Mindset matters. Trust the process. Enjoy the practice.

LISTEN TO YOUR GUT

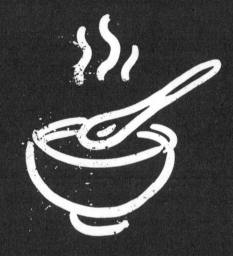

CHAPTER 5

King's Disease

You have to cleanse to heal.
—*Your colon*

In 1939, England's King George and Queen Elizabeth visited Canada. A Canadian whiskey entrepreneur saw this as an opportunity and took advantage of the royal visit to craft a whiskey inspired by the royal couple to present to them as a gift.

He made more than six hundred blends before settling on the final product, which consisted of a proprietary blend of over fifty whiskeys bottled in an ornamental glass vessel and dressed in a regal purple cloth bag with gold stitching. He presented the whiskey to the King and Queen and named it *Crown Royal* in their honor.

The word on the streets about the whiskey fit for a king quickly spread, and today it's still the top-selling Canadian whiskey in America. I don't know about you, but I remember how popular it was back in the day in my house, because no matter how many other bottles and brands of liquor that stood as staples on countertops around our crib—and there were plenty—my pops always kept him some Crown Royal in that iconic purple sack. As a small boy, if you're lucky enough to have your father in your life, whatever you see them do—bad, good, or whatever—it leaves an impression on you.

And then crack happened.

The '80s crack epidemic devastated my family. I was traumatized. I saw firsthand how crazy shit gets messing with drugs, 'cause I watched my big brother get kicked out the house and end up addicted to crack cocaine as a teenager. My pops, his friends, my cousins, people all around the neighborhood were on drugs and suffering. Our kingdom was crumbling. I promised myself I would never even take a sip of alcohol, and I meant it!

But I remember the night I broke that promise.

I was hanging out one weekend with my cuzzo Mario (rest in peace) and a few other cousins, and he asked me to ride out with them to go to this pool party at some chick's crib. We all piled into his maroon Monte Carlo and pulled up on the apartment complex. 'Rio parked a little ways down from the pool area where people were already enjoying themselves, cut off the car, and turned off the headlights.

I was sitting in the backseat between two of my other cousins, looking out the window at the turquoise glow of the pool, when Mario turned around from the driver's seat and said, "Cuz, you don't never drink, you don't get down with the boys, man, you're a square."

Classic peer pressure.

Mario was ten toes down in the street life, and he had long been trying to influence me to get "down" with the code. For years I had been exposed to all kinds of street shit, but I had held my ground and been like, "Man, I'm peer-pressure proof, you can't after-school special me! Y'all do what y'all do but I ain't messing with none of that shit." They would tease me and call me Malcolm X. They probably saw me like Sharif in *Menace II Society,* leaning on the cooler kicking his self-righteous sermon about why we shouldn't be using the white man's poisons.

But that particular night, I was maybe sixteen or seventeen, and

I think I was just feeling the heaviness of my life and I wanted some relief, some escape. On top of that, I was feeling what I couldn't have defined at the time, but I've since learned is social anxiety, about going to the party, 'cause I would often get shy in crowds of people I didn't know. I was tired of all my insecurities. I was tired of being the square peg. I was tired of feeling like an outsider in my own family. Right or wrong, I just wanted to belong and feel accepted. So, when I heard the cap seal crack open on one of the thirty-two-ounce bottles of malt liquor Mario was about to start passing around, I shocked everybody.

"Man, give me that shit," I said, and I started chugging that motherfucker to the face!

Now, if you have any experience with malt liquor, you know it don't take but a few swallows of that bittersweet carbonation to start feeling that buzz. In that moment, I was feeling all these bubbling and tingling sensations in my mind and body, and I was liking it. I kept gulping Louis Armstrong–looking cheeks full of beer, and my cuzzins are laughing and cheering me on. Giving in to the pressure didn't feel so bad. I was feeling a rush of energy like I had never felt before, feeling like one of the guys. By the time I got to the bottom of the bottle, I was lit up! It was like I drank a magic potion that made the insecure me invisible and made my alter ego come to the surface. I was in a "let's fucking go" state of mind, a whole different state of consciousness. It felt amazing!

We hit up the party, and I had the time of my life! I was out-of-my-mind drunk but functional. I felt so confident. I was charming the ladies, whispering whatever silly shit came to my mind in random girls' ears, and they were eating it up. I was high-fiving strangers. Stumbling and bumping into people. Throwing back plastic red cups full of whatever 'Rio and them was sipping. I was dancing and having a blast. The positive feedback from my cousins put the battery in my back that much more. They were enjoying me in this new mood as much as I was. I was so wet that night I almost fell in the fucking swimming pool!

Before the next weekend even rolled around, I found myself feeling like I wanted to have that feeling again. And so of course that's what happened, and then that turned into every weekend. Then every weekend turned into every day. Whenever I wanted to escape, I found it.

It got to where I was the drink champ of the crew—nobody went harder than me. I'm talking blackout drunk.

One minute I'd be thinking I'm just enjoying my buzz off cocktails at random house parties with the homies, music lit, glasses clinking, dro in the air, and the next thing I knew I'd wake up butt naked in the bathroom with vomit everywhere. That became a pattern in my teens. When I moved to New York, I was maybe twenty and my tolerance was even higher by then, but I'd still black out there, too.

We'd get wet before we went to the clubs and then get even more bent once we were seated at our table. Me and the crew would be having the time of our lives, throwing back round after round of shots, and then all of a sudden, I'd cross the point of no return and boom—I'd wake up wasted and slobbering while being pulled from under the table.

I would drink Olde E, Ballantine's, E&J, Henny, Heineken, André, really whatever was clever, but do you know what had a special place on my shelf? That purple sack of Crown Royal.

A Royal Pain

I was living in the county of Kings, Fort Greene in Brooklyn to be specific, and the world-famous *Junior's* restaurant was one of my favorite local spots to hang and bang. Located on the corner of Flatbush and DeKalb Avenues in downtown Brooklyn, just stumbling distance up the street from my one-bedroom apartment on Ashland Place, the iconic old-school neighborhood diner with its rusty-orange booth seating and red-and-white-striped menus is world renowned for its cheesecake and other comfort-food delights. Everyone from Kuwaiti princes to presidents, and even a dead president or two, like myself, has made it a point to indulge at the local landmark.

I indulged a lot. One particular late night, around 3:00 a.m., I was there by myself wolfing down a huge plate of chicken parmesan and steak fries. I'd probably had about four or five blunts by then, easily, and was washing it all down with a second or maybe a third double-rum piña colada. Way over my fill, I tipped the waitress, slid out of my usual booth, and wobbled my drunk ass across Flatbush Avenue and down Fulton Street to my apartment just a short walk away. Like a drunken master, somehow I stayed on my feet, found my keys, and got inside my spot to pass out facedown on the futon.

A few hours later, I woke up to use the bathroom. Still half asleep—still drunkish—I expected to step out of bed onto the cold hardwood floor. Instead, it felt like I had stepped in fire—and the pain was so sudden and intense that I fell flat on my face. I pushed myself up and sat there in the twilight on the floor, so shocked I didn't know if I'd been shot, bitten by one of the rats in our building, or if I had just landed wrong and snapped my ankle. When I got up and limped to turn on the light and looked closer my ankle was red and swollen. Something was definitely wrong.

Afya rushed over, and after taking one look at the swelling, she was like, "You need to go to the doctor, ASAP!" Of course, like a lot of folks I had no doctor to go to and no health insurance to pay for it, either. But after calling around, Afya helped me find a doc who would see me as a walk-in.

The visit was brief, but it was life changing.

"Do you drink alcohol?" doc asked. "Do you smoke? Do you eat a lot of meat? Fast foods? Fried foods?"

I'm like "What, is he psychic?" Of course, the answer was, "Yup, all of the above."

"You have gout," doc pronounced.

Gout. *Gout?*

I thought to myself, "Ain't gout what I used to hear church ladies with fat ankles complaining about? Gout is some old people shit. I'm too young. How *I* got gout?"

Back in the day, gout was literally considered a royal pain. Thousands of years before Nas named his album *King's Disease* after the ailment, gout was first diagnosed and described in ancient Egypt in 2640 BC. It came to be known as "the disease of kings" because only the most rich and powerful could afford a diet that was gluttonous enough in meats and alcohol to trigger gout pain. European royalty appear to have been disproportionately afflicted by the disease. The Roman emperor Charles V, also known as King Charles I of Spain, suffered from gout. King Henry VIII was famous for his gluttony, and gout and obesity contributed to his death at the age of fifty-five. While writing this book, I learned my father had gout in his late thirties.

But at the time, I was only twenty-one.

Doc explained that gout develops from too much uric acid getting in the bloodstream, which I realized, in my case, came from my regular blackout-level alcohol binges. Not to mention the toxic diet that I was living off of—comfort food, fried food, fast food, and junk food—pretty much the standard American hood diet everywhere. Chainsmoking Dutch Masters and White Owl blunts didn't help either. He said that uric acid crystallizes in the blood like tiny slivers of glass. Unhealthy habits and lifestyle choices like mine led to a buildup of toxins, and because I wasn't giving my body the opportunity to process or flush them, they got stuck in and around the joints—wrists, fingers, knees, heels, and toes. In my case, it happened in my ankle and that's what caused the super painful swelling.

I just wanted to know how to get rid of it.

The doc said, "You don't get rid of it, because there's no known cure. You manage it."

And then, like doctors get paid to do, he proceeded to write me a prescription for some drugs. He told me that when my condition flared back up, the drugs he prescribed might be able to soften the stabbing sensations and maybe help the symptoms disappear faster.

"Damn, that's the best you can do, Doc? I just got to be on meds from now on?"

I was tight.

I left the doctor's office with Afya feeling like I was in a bad dream. I didn't want to be on no medication for the rest of my life. And I didn't trust doctors—or the American health-care system—anyways. I didn't know what I was going to do.

Out on the sidewalk, Afya had a radical idea. I've never forgotten those words. "Babe," she said, "I believe in the body's ability to heal itself if we give it the proper tools."

Afya and I first met when she was eighteen and I was nineteen. She was *woke* long before that was a popular term. She was a beautiful, smart engineering major at Florida A&M University, which happened to be in my hometown of Tallahassee, and I was a local hoodster, thuggin in the streets, pimping the system every way I could, one of which was taking advantage of the resources and connections on campus though I never actually enrolled. We met at a revolutionary themed poetry event I was guest hosting on campus, and we hit it off immediately. She told me that everything went black when she saw me onstage, as if there were a spotlight just on me and everything else around me faded. Something told her she had to meet me. When she came up to me, I could feel the "I'm digging you" vibes she was sending me. Her natural beauty; clear golden skin; long, healthy black hair; big, beautiful eyes; cute dimples and amazing smile; and the eclectic denim ensemble she was rocking all had me like, "Damn she is fine, and earthy, and different!" She reminded me of Freddy from the hit *Cosby Show* spin-off, *A Different World*. From that night on, we were like two peas in a pod for many, many years to come.

The name *Afya* is a Kiswahili term that means "healthy."

After getting to know her a lot more from our deep all-night conversations, I found out she had plenty of experience under her belt in natural healing because she had been through her own health challenges growing up sickly with asthma, irritable bowel syndrome, and a host of allergies. She had been on medication after medication and had to take painful shots all the time. By the time she was a teen, she was tired of taking pills and getting shots and she was still suffering under the Western medical approach. By going vegetarian she was able to heal herself and reduce her symptoms. Afya was the most health-conscious person I knew personally at the time, and I trusted her instincts when, standing outside of that doctor's office, she said, "We're going to go all the way vegan."

"Fuck it," I said. "Vegan it is. Let's do it."

I never got the prescription the doc gave me filled. Instead, over the next few weeks I went through a total dietary transformation that ultimately changed the trajectory of my life.

Afya immediately put me on a detox program: lots of dark leafy-green salads, mad water, and fresh fruits and green vegetable juices. She had me drink tart cherry juice to help reduce the inflammation in my ankle. No more meat, no eggs, no cheese. No sodas or any other sugary drinks; anything that wasn't water or fresh juice was off-limits. Processed ingredients like white sugar and white flour—white bread—were all out. All the greasy Styrofoam takeout containers of Chinese chicken and broccoli—outta here. No more one-dollar pizza slices. No KFC, no Mickey D's, no Burger King. If it wasn't a real, whole food from the plant kingdom, it was off-limits. I gave up alcohol cold turkey, too. It was a drastic shift from everything I was used to.

But sometimes a drastic change can set you up for a major come-up.

Smai Tawi: Disease Begins in the Colon

Health is a golden crown, placed on the brow of the healthy that only the sick can see.

—*Ancient Egyptian proverb*

As part of my healing regimen, Afya put me on to the Brooklyn-based Queen Afua, a world-renowned holistic healer, best-selling author, and owner and director of the Smai Tawi Heal Thyself/ Know Thyself Afrakan Wellness and Kultural Center. Smai Tawi is based on the African tradition of Kemetic yoga. In Kemetic yoga, not only are there physical postures, breathing techniques, and spiritual tenets, but enlightened nutritional practices and self-healing are also very much a part of the package. Queen Afua was instrumental in my healing process, beginning when she taught me the theory that disease begins in the colon and recommended a series of colonics at the center.

A colonic is a natural healing procedure where an infusion of water is pumped through a tube into the rectum to flush out the colon and the large intestine. Also called colonic hydrotherapy or colon irrigation, the process is effective for clearing our guts of backed-up waste and toxins.

Colon hydrotherapy has been around for thousands of years in many cultures from Mesopotamia, China, India, Native American tribes, the Essenes, and others, but the oldest known iteration of the gut-cleansing process was in the form of enemas as mentioned as early as 1550 BC in an Egyptian medical document called the "Ebers Papyrus." The process was considered so much a part of good health to the ancient Egyptians that the pharaohs actually created an official position in their court called the "shepherd of the anus" whose job it was to personally administer the pharaoh's enemas. The writings attribute the inspiration for the use of this method to maintain the pharaoh's health to the god-king Ausar—a metaphor for the principle of regeneration, personified—who observed an ibis bird that was in a river, filling its beak with water and inserting and releasing the water back into its own butt.

But everybody ain't have their own ass shepherd. The common folk gave themselves enemas in rivers. They'd use a hollow reed to channel water to flow into the rectum. The Greeks got hip to the Egyptian game and then people like Hippocrates, Herodotus, and others started to advocate the practice in their writings and teachings. In the late 1400s, King Louis XI credited enemas with relieving his seizures. A later king, Louis XIII, received over two hundred enemas in one year. Another king, Louis XIV, reportedly had over two thousand enemas during his reign. He even held meetings with members of his court during the procedure. A wild boy. It wasn't until the 1800s that the invention of rubber led to a comfortable rubber nozzle that made enemas much easier and effective to use. Over time, the invention of a colonic machine revolutionized the process.

By the early 1900s, Dr. John H. Kellogg believed that 90 percent of all disease in the human body results from the improper functioning of the colon. He developed his theory from the research he performed using colon hydrotherapy on over forty thousand patients. He reported in the *Journal of the American Medical Association* that in all but twenty cases, he used no surgery for the treatment of gastrointestinal disease in his patients; they were instead healed by the cleansing of the bowel, improved diet, and exercise.

Queen Afua assured me that colonics were not only safe and effective but also essential for the deep healing I needed at the time. I reasoned, what could be better for a king's disease than a queen's cure?

So, I agreed to the royal flush.

But dawg, trust me when I tell you, it was no fun.

You lay on your side and a colon therapist puts a narrow tube a few centimeters in your butt and starts filling you up with warm water. It feels weird as hell; your stomach expands until it feels like it's about to pop. Then the therapist removes the tube, and you hurry your ass off that table and go plop down on the toilet because all that water and all your backed-up shit is on its way back out with a vengeance!

And that's just round one.

All in all, I did around six of them bad boys over a series of sessions.

I hated it every time.

But in just a few weeks, with my new diet heavy on the veggies and a squeaky-clean gastrointestinal tract, guess what?

No more gout.

And it's never come back once, after all these years.

If I would have listened to that doctor, I would probably still be on meds or worse. But I listened to my gut and found a natural way to heal. I knew I didn't have to be on medication for the rest of my life. Afya said the body can heal itself when given the proper tools, and I trusted her instincts. Experiencing that truth in my own body made it super real for me. As a young king learning more and more about alternative healing and holistic health, the whole experience was adding jewel after jewel to my crown.

I BELIEVE IN THE BODY'S ABILITY TO HEAL ITSELF
IF GIVEN THE PROPER TOOLS.

—AFYA IBOMU

Crown Heights

My natural healing process turned out to be more than a diet change. It set off a personal revolution. This was years before eating vegan would become a popular, mainstream thing. There was no nut milk latte option at the coffee shop, no meat-free burgers on restaurant menus; the only fake meats available in those days were in specialty health-food stores—slimy, disgusting vegan Vienna sausages in a can. If you were vegan in those days, it was slim pickings! And if you weren't at the very edge of the frontier, it just wouldn't be on your radar.

I got lucky. I left my old apartment in Fort Greene and the new neighborhood I moved into turned out to be the perfect environment for all these new healthier shifts to become deeply rooted in my way of living. This new neighborhood was none other than the one and only Crown Heights, planet Brooklyn—and at times it really did feel like another planet. Back then, Crown Heights was leading the pack in kindling its own revolutionary world of Black health consciousness.

I attended early local lectures and gatherings held by triple OGs from the natural healing community like Dr. Sebi, Dr. Afrika, Dr. Aris LaTham, Ra Un Nefer Amen, and many others. These folks were continuing the healing work that's always been part of the Black experience since we arrived on these shores (and thousands of years before)—healthy, community-based practices and information exchange that continued through the food and breakfast programs of the Black Panther Survival Programs in the '60s and '70s and the awareness raising of health-focused icons in the '70s like comedian Dick Gregory and others.

So, as I was cleansing and detoxing my body in my new hood with new ways of eating and healing, my hood was also feeding my crown, with nutrient-dense food for thought for healthy living.

I started meeting more and more people who were vegans with powerful testimonies about the power of plant-based living. There were Muslim shops with halal buffets and juice bars, raw foodists, fruitarians, pescatarians, and more. But of all the various schools of thought in the mix that I encountered in those days, I think the most influential to me, on multiple levels, were the Rastas.

Roots and Culture

Where Afya and I lived in the Heights, on Nostrand Avenue and Dean Street, was smack-dab in the middle of a powerful Rastafarian community where all the vibrant vibes of the movement—which was originated in the Maroon hills of Jamaica and was popularized around the world by Bob Marley and reggae music—came to life on the New York City streets.

There were Rasta-owned record shops with huge speakers positioned along the sidewalks blasting the best of reggae old and new, day in and day out. In reggae culture, there's a dynamic of ghetto-rude-boy and righteous-roots-man coexisting in a natural yin and yang, which I felt right at home in. I was learning to understand and appreciate the powerful poetry in the patois that was chatted in and sung on the dance-hall mixtapes and vintage-roots records. The melodies, the messages, it all moved me: Sizzla, Steel Pulse, Hugh Mundell, Bob Marley, The Wailers, Jacob Miller, Dennis Brown, so many legends. It was like discovering hip-hop again for the first time. Afya and I watched the cult-classic reggae movie *Rockers* and absolutely fell in love with the styles and the vibes and the soundtrack. It was like the soundtrack of our new life!

Even though veganism, as we know it today, was just in its infancy, Crown Heights had lots of vegetarian-friendly Caribbean eateries, raw juice bars, and Rasta-owned "bush medicine" herbal apothecaries back in the nineties. There was an African-centered vegan buffet called Imhotep's; a pescatarian Rasta spot called Veggie Seafood; Tony's Country Life, a Trinidadian-owned herbal supplement shop; Sister Kutchie's spot with her signature roots drinks; and a few other late-night pop-up Rasta shops that would serve hearty stews and veggie patties. I "reasoned" with the local bredren daily. There were lean and lanky gold-toothed hustlers with long, thick locs wrapped up in bundles on top of their heads, with sharp cutlasses for opening coconuts and cutting stalks of sugarcane that they sold along the sidewalks. We could stroll the block and eat Trinidadian coco bread, rotis stuffed with pumpkin and chickpeas, Jamaican callaloo patties, rice and peas with a slice of pear (how Jamaicans refer to avocado), a hearty Ital stew and dumplings, or sweet plantains, and wash it all down sipping on a fresh-cut coconut from one block to the next.

The whole scene nourished me every day.

Rastas don't always get the credit they deserve for their influence on the shift to healthier lifestyles in the Black community and beyond. They're known worldwide for their deep reverence for cannabis as a sacrament and a medicinal herb, but I also witnessed Rastas in my neighborhood emphasizing a set of holistic, nutritional, and lifestyle values called Ital, Rasta vernacular for vital. Long before the British woodworker Donald Watson coined the term "vegan" in 1944 to distinguish people who were vegetarian but who also did not eat dairy and eggs, there was Ital. Ital food is almost always plant-based, nutritious ground food. Sometimes, in some circles, fish is included, but the emphasis is always toward natural and pure without chemical additives or preservatives, or even too much salt. The Rasta Ital way of living, or "Livity" as it's referred to in the culture, was promoting plant-based living before that was even a term. Rasta culture is an OG in healthy living and a rich source of wisdom and experience on living simply and naturally—especially in urban environments.

Jewel in the Crown

On the day Afya and I moved into the basement apartment of the three-story brownstone that would become our home for the next seven years, I found an abandoned tam-style cap woven in the Rasta Ethiopian flag colors of red, green, and gold on the ground. It felt like a sign or something, so I picked it up, washed it, and kept it as my own to rock on my newly growing locs. Before long, my bushy 'fro was filling up that cap, naturally coiling and clumping into unpredictable nappy clusters like a wild forest. Influenced by the organic beauty of the Rasta community in Crown Heights, after a lifetime of fresh haircuts, I just let my hair free up and nap up, wild style, and so did Afya. Neither of us wanted the beauty-shop styled locs; we wanted the "Nyahbingi" free-form locs where you let your hair just do what it do.

The Black, Creole, and Native roots of Afya's naturally curly hair bloomed into big, beautiful locs in no time. She also started crocheting and selling her own tams. Crocheting was a skill Afya learned from her grandmother and mom. She named her custom crochet business *Who the Cap Fit*, after the Bob Marley song, and I drew the logo tags—a happy, nappy couple, both rocking colorful tams. It was a big hit in the neighborhood and in our artsy extended circle. The homies Common, Talib, Black Thought, Sway, Musiq Soulchild, Badu, and many others supported us by buying many of her hats in those early days. In fact, that's how we met Erykah Badu when she and Common were dating. He brought her by the crib one day to pick up a batch of hats Afya made for him, and we all became friends.

Badu was really into natural health too, so we clicked in that area as well. She would put us on to all kinds of healthy jewels. She made herbal tea for us when we'd visit her Brooklyn apartment and hang out and vibe with her and Common. She laid out royal spreads of vegan delights while we visited her during her studio sessions at Electric Lady in Manhattan. She had these little packets of Sun Chlorella powder, spirulina tablets, and liquid chlorophyll drops that she'd add to her water and it would turn green. We double dated with her and Common at local veggie spots. The green crocheted tam that Badu rocks on her *Mama's Gun* album cover is one of many that Afya made for her. The craftsmanship, colors, and creativity of Afya's crowns really embodied the inspiration we were absorbing in Crown Heights. It was the hood, no doubt, but also a healthy, beautiful, authentic community we called home.

A Whole New Life

Afya and I had been together about seven years; we were deeply in love. Around this time, I toured South Africa with dead prez and other groups like the Roots, Black Star, and the Coup. This was a very special trip for me—it was my first time ever visiting Africa, so I brought Afya along because I didn't want to experience the motherland without her.

While in Botswana, Afya experienced a lot of nausea. We thought she might have gotten a bug from the water or something, but no—to my surprise and our delight, she was pregnant. Afya had always been adamant about her faith in natural home birth, and I was with that 100 percent. She was also determined to remain vegan during the pregnancy. We hired Taioma, a doula who came highly recommended in our conscious community network. Afya and I started taking tai chi classes together as a form of Lamaze to prepare for a peaceful and healthy delivery. Badu was a great help during the pregnancy. She had one of her assistants who lived in Brooklyn, the homey, Revolution, deliver Afya a green juice damn near every day of the nine months of her pregnancy.

Afya's water broke on a sunny Sunday afternoon at the beginning of June. Her mom and sister and a few of her close friends came over to support the home-birth process with Taioma. Badu was supposed to be on a flight and changed her plans to come be bedside in our basement apartment for the birth. She brought her acoustic guitar and sang songs to Afya's belly while we all awaited the big moment. And man did we wait. Hours went by.

The sun went down and came back up the next day on Monday, and still no baby.

Every hour the anticipation grew more intense. We were doing all the things our midwife instructed: walks, massages, and being patient. But the baby wasn't ready to come. It was frustrating. At one point, Afya went into the bathroom and locked herself in there and wouldn't respond to any of us. I felt worried, and as tears rolled down my cheeks, I realized in the deepest way that as much as I wanted to protect her and our child, I was not in control.

Afya finally came out of the bathroom and said she just needed a moment to be by herself with the baby and make peace with allowing the birth to happen. There were heavy emotions for us all.

But as time dripped by, nearing the end of Monday with almost forty-eight hours in labor and still no baby, things got critical. Taioma pulled me off to the side and said, "Dad, we need to talk. I know Afya does *not* want to deliver that baby in the hospital. But if *you* don't do something, I'm going to have to recommend we go to the hospital and have the doctors induce labor." She said, "I know she don't wanna go, but she's gonna have to go if you don't do something."

If I don't do something? I thought to myself, I ain't no midwife, I don't know shit about delivering no baby. Ain't that what you're here for? What am I supposed to do? But then a deep silence and stillness came over me, and I knew I had to just follow my gut instinct. I said to Taioma, "Alright," and walked into our bedroom and gathered everyone next to Afya as she laid on our futon bed.

I took Afya's hand and led her to stand up in a squatting position like Kunte Kinte's mama stood when she was giving birth to him in the movie *Roots*. The tribe all circled around her holding hands. Instinctively, I started letting out a noise that was like a deep exhale and a yell at the same time.

"Aaaaahhhhh!" I said loudly and slowly.

Again. "Aaaaahhhhh!" and everyone joined in.

All together—"Aaaaaaaaaah!"

Afya, her sister and mom, Taioma, Badu, a few other friends, and I, we all kept repeating the chant:

"Aaaaaaaaaahhhhhh!"

And then all of a sudden, I hear Taioma yell out, "I see the crown! Keep going!"

Finally, on Tuesday, June 5, after fifty-two hours of labor and one of the bravest, boldest, and most beautiful things I've ever witnessed Afya do, our first child was born right there into my hands in our basement apartment. Bright, regal eyes, wide open, looking around at everyone, peaceful, calm, and very alert. No crying at all. Tai chi classes must have worked, I thought, because this little Zen master came out in super-chill mode. Taioma washed our baby clean and I cut the umbilical cord. Afya's mom was supposed to be filming the whole thing but she got so caught up in the excitement she forgot all about turning the camera on. I was so dazed and amazed that it hadn't even occurred to me what the sex was until our friend Wubnesh (may she rest in peace) yelled out, "It's a boy!"

Supremely grateful and extremely exhausted, I laid my young prince against my chest and we both passed out.

Having witnessed firsthand the power of a healthy, nourishing environment with the safe and natural arrival of my son, it got me deeply reflecting on the larger environment we live in.

Hunger Games

When a potted plant isn't growing and thriving you don't blame the plant, you check the soil.

All the positive seeds that were sprouting in my life going through all the healthy transformations got me thinking about all the unhealthy indoctrination I grew up surrounded by—the conventional food pyramid that was pushed on us in school and how it promoted eating mad meat, eggs, and dairy products even though the leading cause of death in the US population is heart disease, and Black and brown communities are largely lactose intolerant.

Make it make sense.

I was asking questions like: Why is it that in most hoods, it always be junk food–filled bodegas and corner stores, fast-food restaurants and liquor stores on damn near every corner, but fresh fruits and veggies be so few and far between? Was this planned?

You already know it was—city planning don't happen randomly. Any community, from a small country town to sprawling urban metropolis, is built based on extensive and strategic planning.

In big cities, the department of city planning prepares the master development strategy in a thorough physical document, sometimes hundreds of pages long, that shows a detailed agenda for what a community will be like ten, fifteen, twenty years in advance. The plans contain extensive research, reports, and statistical information that's gathered to support the intended vision. We often say that's just how shit is when we look at our communities, but the shit ain't just happening how it is by itself for no reason. No cities just happen to be how they are; the conditions come to be the way they are by deliberate design. You don't see certain liquor stores and fast-food restaurants and convenience stores in wealthier neighborhoods, yet you see them all over the place in the hood. From city to city and state to state, you see the same patterns—lower-income zoned neighborhoods get the unhealthy options and higher-income zip codes get the healthier options. That's not accidental.

I also thought about all the unhealthy messages we receive through TV commercials, marketed to our eyeballs and taste buds for profit with no regard to the effects these products have on people's lives. I thought about how holidays like Thanksgiving and Christmas hijack the sentiment of spending quality time with our families and instead indoctrinate generation after generation with poor dietary habits, unhealthy cravings, and addictions celebrated as cultural traditions in our communities.

As delicious as it was, I began to make the connection between the typical Southern soul-food diet I grew up on and the three heart attacks my dad suffered, which resulted in several metal stents surgically inserted in his heart to keep his arteries open. I remembered how my mom developed diabetes and had to inject herself with insulin shots every day because her body could no longer properly regulate the excessive sugar in her bloodstream.

In the environment that I was born and raised in, terrible eating habits were as convenient as the sugar cubes in those monkey traps I mentioned earlier. We have easy access to what we have been conditioned to crave, but at what price?

I'm grateful for the sacrifices my mom and dad made to put food on the table no matter what level of health awareness they had; I'm appreciative and I know the intention was in the right place, and I know my parents meant what was best. Some people had nothing to eat, so for the fact that I had food to eat at all, healthy or not, I'm thankful and grateful. With that said, in terms of *health*, the truth is, even when the love and good intentions are there, so many of us are still exposed to too much of the wrong stuff, too much of the time, and don't get nearly enough of the good stuff enough of the time.

As I kept reflecting, reading, researching, and learning more and more, I started to feel like Neo in *The Matrix*. In the first offering of the classic sci-fi trilogy, Neo's mentor Morpheus gave him the option of taking one of two pills. If he chose the blue pill, he could just go back to sleep and return to blissful ignorance. The red pill meant remaining aware of all of life's unpleasant and uncomfortable truths.

For me, the blue pill would have been getting the doctor's prescription filled, and I'm sure eventually resorting back to the same old negative patterns I was familiar with. However, a total plant-based transformation, the "red pill" that Afya proposed, offered an opportunity to take the power into my own hands and learn how to heal myself naturally.

I chose the red pill.

Healthy Is the New Gangsta

Clearing my body of gout was a huge victory for me and it inspired me to imagine winning even bigger battles. I began to wonder what my life would be like if I dedicated myself to living healthy with the same level of intensity I had when living an unhealthy lifestyle. What if I went hard drinking water like I had been drinking alcohol? Instead of going back to the bullshit I was used to, why couldn't healthy be my new gangsta? How far could I take it? Health couldn't be a bad investment! How awesome would it feel to dedicate my life to well-being? I was inspired just imagining what the quality of my life might turn out to be if I stayed on this healthy wave for the long haul.

I thought about the positive impact I might have on my homies if the guy that was always one of the wildest cannons in the crew and the drunkest in the room made a 180-degree turnaround.

Also, somewhere in the back of my mind, I hoped that my transformation might even help or rub off on my big brother in some way

WHO KNOWS WHAT'S GOOD OR BAD?

There was an old, wise farmer. Every day, he relied on his only horse to help him do the hard work of managing a farm. One day, the horse up and ran away. Some of the neighbors in his village heard the news and came by and said, "We're so sorry to hear your horse left, sorry for the bad news."

and inspire him to get off drugs and get his life back to a healthy place.

Some people might see a debilitating disease like gout as a failure or a sign to give up. But my experience with gout had a positive impact on me because the physical pain and the shock of the diagnosis broke the spell that my negative habits had on me. It opened my mind to consider the radical changes that I so needed to make. And dig it: until I started experiencing revolutionary changes in my own mind and body, I had believed that the whole world—including the unjust and oppressive political system—would have to change before anything that I did would make a difference. Taking my health into my own hands put me in touch with my own personal power and a feeling of liberation that I didn't expect. I didn't have to wait for change to happen around me; I could start being the change I needed—immediately!

That diagnosis of king's disease was a blessing in disguise. I had been sleeping on the power of nutrition and taking my health for granted, as so many of us unconsciously do, but gout created an opportunity for me to fix my crown, take charge of my health, grow and change, and break that pattern. I saw that if my toxic habits and harmful choices had enough power to put me in a state of personal crisis and illness, then staying committed to a healthier lifestyle would help keep me in a state of vitality and wellness.

But the farmer responded, "Who knows what's good or bad?"

Time went by, and then one afternoon, while the farmer was working outside, he looked up and saw his horse running toward him. But the horse was not alone. It was followed by a whole herd of horses. In that time, if any animal was on your land, you automatically became the owner, so now the farmer had ten horses to help work his fields.

The neighbors came by again to congratulate the farmer and said, "Wow! This is such good news!"

But the farmer simply responded, "Who knows what's good or bad?"

A few weeks later, the farmer's oldest son was helping work on the farm. While trying to tame one of the wild horses, the farmer's son fell and cracked his shinbone in two.

The villagers came by once again. "How terrible. This is such bad luck."

But as he always replied, the farmer calmly responded, "Who knows what's good or bad?"

A couple weeks later, the farmer's son was, of course, still recovering, and so was still unable to walk or do any manual labor to help out around the farm.

That's when, all of a sudden, a regiment of the King's army came marching through the local village. The king had declared war to expand the territory of the empire and the soldiers were there for an immediate and mandatory draft of every able-bodied young man to join them in war. When the troops came to the farmer's house and saw his son's broken leg, they just marched right past him and moved on to the next village.

The Wisdom in Our Wounds

Your body is the temple of knowledge.

—*African proverb*

Once again, the villagers came over to say "Wow, it was so fortunate that your son wasn't drafted for war. You have such good luck."

And you already know what the farmer's response was…

"Who knows what's good or bad?"

The things that happen in our lives are not necessarily good or bad, because they are not isolated events, they are part of a continuum. When things seem to go according to our plans, in the moment, we judge them as good. But when things don't turn out as we might have preferred in a given moment, we judge events as bad.

But as the story of the wise farmer shows us, we don't always know whether an event will ultimately prove to be "good" or "bad."

When I was first diagnosed with gout, it felt like I was in a bad predicament, but as things unfolded, it was actually one of the best things that could've happened to me because it helped me become much healthier.

So, I've learned to try to be more like the wise farmer and withhold my judgment of whether events in my life are good or bad, and just roll with things with an attitude that within all the challenges life throws at us there are advantages and opportunities.

We each have powerful innate mechanisms for self-healing that help us maintain or reestablish the natural balance of our bodily functions, which is known as homeostasis. It ain't the doctor that *heals* you, or the drugs. The body is able to fully regenerate itself. When you injure yourself, maybe you have a wound from a bad cut, there are four stages you progress through en route to healing. The technical names for these four stages are: hemostasis (not to be confused with homeostasis), inflammation, proliferation, and maturation.

Hemostasis literally means to "stop the bleeding," but more generally speaking, it implies that you have to first stop doing whatever is causing the damage.

In the second phase of healing—inflammation—the body sounds an alarm and starts to try and contain the damage. The uncomfortable, painful swelling we experience as inflammation is actually a red-alert response of the immune system; white blood cells flood the damaged area to secure the perimeter and start fighting off and preventing any further spread of damage or infection and start getting rid of damaged cells. That pain is actually part of the healing process.

Next, during *proliferation*, the third stage of healing, new cells are pumped in to repair and rebuild. This is the scabbing and remodeling stage.

And the last stage, maturation, is when the new cells have replaced the old, damaged ones and the wounded area is not only repaired and good as new, but it's actually been upgraded—reinforced and fortified to be even more resilient against potential injuries in the future. The skin is much stronger than before. The maturation process can go on for months and even years, and the healed area keeps getting stronger every day.

On a deeper level, we experience these stages in all kinds of healing.

First, we have to stop whatever is causing the damage. In my case, I had to cut out all the bullshit I was doing to myself. I had to realize all the toxic things that were feeding into me were not serving my best interest, and I had to decide to change.

Secondly, we have to understand that the inflammation and pain that we feel is the body communicating where the need to heal is, and we have to cleanse and protect that sensitive area from any further damage while we are nourishing it with helpful things that restore and repair.

For me, that meant detoxing my body, my gut, and my mind, giving my body nourishing foods and water and putting myself in positive environments that influence me in healthy ways.

When we do this, not only are we able to heal what was hurting, but we also become even stronger and resilient in the process. The rite-of-passage journey I went through healing from gout turned me on to so much life-game; it totally transformed my life. I didn't just get back to the state of health I was in before gout, I upgraded my quality of life tenfold!

With all of man's scientific advancements, from intergalactic space travel to quantum physics to sophisticated electrical engineering and artificial intelligence, scientists still don't know how to make a scab. But the body knows. The fact that a cut on your arm heals by itself if allowed to reveals that there is an indwelling intelligence in the body that has incredible knowledge. And that wisdom is ours to tap into. That part of us that knows how to heal is an amazing part of our being. Our wounds hold wisdom just waiting to be discovered. Our bodies speak to us in powerful ways if only we learn how to listen to the body's language.

As we learn to listen and trust that universal voice within, we can hear its subtle whispers and nudges calling us toward necessary and beneficial change.

CHAPTER 6

Plant Forward

Everything changes.
—*Tao Te Ching*

Here's how you know you've officially become a foodie: When food and everything about it becomes a source of inspiration! The culinary arts get you excited like sports do for sports fans. You enjoy trying new cuisines and dishes at new restaurants. You even enjoy shopping for groceries and get excited to try all kinds of new ingredients. You're buying food magazines and cookbooks, excited about being in the kitchen more and nerding out about spices and herbs and different ways to bring more flavor to your cooking. Gardeners and chefs are like rock stars to you; indulging in their cooking philosophies and stories are forms of entertainment. You have fun experimenting when cooking—you don't always rely on recipes, you're adding your own twist and discovering new combinations that you like. When cooking and eating become a cultural exploration and adventure, you've become a bona fide foodie!

After my initiation into the wonderful world of plant-based living, I definitely became a foodie. I maintained a strict vegan diet for ten years. Afya enrolled in the Institute for Integrative Nutrition and earned a professional certification as a Holistic Health Counselor with flying colors, and went on some years after that to earn her bachelor's degree in nutrition from Georgia State. All of her enthusiasm for food and nutrition rubbed off on me in the best ways. We watched all kinds of cooking shows together; the Food Network was our nightly ritual, and Afya broadened my palate by introducing me to all sorts of plant-based items at restaurants and at home. I was the official chief taste tester for many of the recipes she developed for her award-winning cookbooks *The Vegan Remix* and *The Vegan Soulfood Guide to the Galaxy.*

Food & Travel

Out on tour with dead prez, I learned to appreciate and enjoy all sorts of international plant-based cuisines and cultures and got really good at finding nutritious food that was suitable for my lifestyle no matter where our tour stopped next. If you're working on eating healthier while traveling or just when eating out in general, I figured out a variety of cuisines that are reliable.

You can always count on Thai food to get you right: with a simple side of rice and either a tom kha gai (coconut soup) or a tom yum (spicy tomato soup), you usually can't go wrong.

Chinese restaurants will almost always have steamed or sautéed veggies and rice and some kind of stir-fried tofu offering.

Ethiopian cuisine is one of my all-time favorites in the world, and it's also the oldest cuisine in the world. You can always order the veggie combo. The classic medley of veggies comes with delicious dishes like dark leafy greens (gomen), green beans (fusili), yellow and red lentils (yekik eletcha or ater), all spooned in a circular arrangement on a delicious, spongy fermented bread called injera that serves as an edible plate.

Indian food is another great option. Their lentil (dal) soups and peppery, lemony mulligatawny soups are amazing. You can get tasty chickpea (chana) masala dishes, fragrant cauliflower dishes, and hearty potato and green pea entrées that are rich in layers of flavor and heat!

Being plant based definitely does not limit you to fries and salads. There are so many nutritious and delicious dishes to choose from when you explore different ethnic cuisines. The key to enjoying eating out more is to treat it like an adventure, take an interest in new cultures, ask questions, get recommendations, and try new things.

Going In Raw

At home, I also experimented a lot with simple, quick-to-whip-up raw-food recipes. I even learned to make (and not bake) raw pies. At one point, I went on an eighty-four-day raw-food cleanse; I drank a gang of water every day and I didn't eat no cooked food at all for that three-month period. I discovered a new appreciation for the natural, uncooked, and unprocessed flavors in fresh vegetables, fruits, herbs, nuts, spices, and salads. I went absolutely ham on almond butters! All I needed to be in snack heaven was a bag of apples and a jar of almond butter and you couldn't tell me I wasn't in the lap of luxury! Raw foods are hydrating; they are full of nutrients and live enzymes that help aid digestion. It's always good to incorporate some fresh raw veggies and fruits into our eating regimen, unless you have digestive issues—in that case, raw foods can sometimes be problematic for the gut. Don't force yourself to do anything your body can't handle!

All the insights I had been gaining from vegan living were impacting and changing my life in every way—changes I rapped about on the dead prez record "*Be Healthy*":

They say you are what you eat
So I strive to eat healthy
My goal in life is not to be rich or wealthy
'Cause true wealth comes from good health

And wise ways

We got to start taking better care of ourselves

I rarely, if ever, got sick. But then, after almost a decade of dedication, I started having some little issues.

COOK UP! RAW APPLE PIE WITH DATE-NUT CRUST

I used to make this joint in NYC all the time. When you want a healthy sweet treat, this will get you right, fam. And the crust is nutty—literally. There's no baking or cooking involved. It's made with all raw, vegan, gluten-free, whole-food ingredients and no processed sugar, flour, or dairy.

Prep time: 15 minutes   Makes 1 (9-inch) pie

---

10 to 12 Brazil nuts (or about ¾–1 cup almonds, walnuts, peanuts, or whatever you prefer)

5 Medjool dates

1 teaspoon ground cinnamon, plus more for sprinkling

3 or 4 organic apples (any kind)

Juice of ¼ organic lemon

Blend the nuts, dates, and ¾ teaspoon of the cinnamon together in a food processor to a consistency similar to mashed potato, but chunkier. Spread the mix in a standard 9-inch pie dish. Cover and refrigerate until time to serve.

Lightly blend the apples, lemon juice, and remaining ¼ teaspoon cinnamon in a food processor. Keep it chunky, not smooth like apple sauce. Pour the mixture into the nut crust and top with a sprinkle of cinnamon. Put the pie in the fridge for about an hour to firm it up. Then you're good to go! Easy as pie!

Body Language

While I was definitely taking better care of myself, I started seeing these dry, itchy areas on my skin, in the folds of my arms and behind my knees. I had never had eczema before and my diet was better than ever, so I couldn't understand why I was getting these patches. After a while it became more and more aggravating, but because everything else felt fine, I just kept on with my life, moisturizing with shea butter and keeping it pushing.

I was in Jamaica on tour. On the first morning of my stay, the sun woke me up early, and I went through my usual rituals before breakfast and then reached for some cereal I had packed for the tour—when I travel for tour out the country, I always check a bag of "just in case" foods, snacks, and beverages since finding healthy food options abroad can be unpredictable.

As I reached into my portable mess hall for a carton of almond milk, my intuition spoke to me.

"You're allergic to almonds," the voice said.

Hmmm. That's strange, I thought.

I had been drinking a lot of almond milk and eating almond butter like it was going out of style in recent weeks and months. My intuition felt timely, so I decided to chill for a while on everything almond, just to see if it made a difference.

Sure enough, after a few weeks of staying away from almonds the eczema symptoms had vanished.

My theory was I might have developed an allergic response to almonds after drinking so much almond milk and going so hard on those nut butters. The intuition that surfaced in Jamaica was another one of those unexplainable *knowings*. I started eating other nuts instead—Brazil nuts, walnuts, pecans—but after a while the eczema patches started to return.

I was perplexed. Was I allergic to nuts in general? Cutting out nut-based foods as a vegan would mean missing out on a huge source of protein.

Afya and I were discussing possible causes and solutions when my oldest son came in and dropped a gem on us.

"Baba," he said, "maybe you're just allergic to tree nuts. Maybe you can still have peanuts since they're groundnuts. And technically, they're legumes."

Wow! I hadn't thought of the distinction. And sure enough, to this very day, I haven't eaten any tree nuts—just peanuts and coconuts, which aren't strictly "nuts."

Still, the eczema symptoms would leave for a while, then reappear again. It drove me crazy. Finally, Afya put me on an elimination diet; we removed all the known and suspected foods that might have been triggering my immune system and then slowly added them back one by one over the course of several weeks to find out which food was setting things off—catching the offending food red-handed, in a way.

As a vegan, meat and dairy were already out for me, of course, as were alcohol and most processed sugars and sweeteners. For this elimination protocol I removed all supplements and vitamins first. Also on the list were starches: bread and pasta, anything that might be made from grains like wheat, barley, oats, or corn.

The elimination phase took place gradually over two to three weeks, and I pretty much just ate a gang of fruits and green vegetables, rice, herbal teas, and water. Once Afya determined it had been long enough based on no new flare-ups, we started adding foods one-by-one back into my diet every few days.

The whole process took almost six weeks, but the perseverance and the patience were worth it. In the end the culprit was gluten—protein made from wheat. As a dedicated vegan, I was already caught off guard when I had to cut out tree nuts, which I had come to think of as my go-to source of energy and as great snacks. Turns out I needed to drop most of the meat substitutes as well, since at that time they were almost always made from seitan: gluten, the protein of wheat. This was especially disheartening because I loved sandwiches, and since bread and most of the plant-based fake meat alternatives like veggie burgers, hot dogs, sausages, and turkey-like cold cuts that were starting to make their way to the mainstream and becoming more available at supermarkets and restaurants all contained gluten, going gluten free left me with few options. But listening to my gut, once I eliminated wheat products from my diet, the eczema disappeared. For good.

But the whole experience with food allergies left me starting to wonder if my strict vegan diet was as healthy as I once thought it was.

Gut Check

Ra and I became fast friends after Afya met him and his wife at an event and invited them over to hang out. Afya said she felt Ra and I had so much in common she knew we'd hit it off. Ra was from the hood in Arkansas and he had a background as a hustler in the streets, too, but he was also a deep thinker who, at the time, was inspired heavily by the Rasta movement. We both enjoyed having thoughtful conversations about philosophy, psychology, politics, and life. As we started hanging out more and more Ra and his wife also went vegan.

Over time, I watched Ra get super healthy and fit and it was a beautiful transformation to witness. I invited him on dead prez tours, and we'd be hanging, enjoying the best vegan foods, training, and building our friendship. After a while, Ra was really excelling on his regimen and had gotten in like magazine-cover-model shape. His wife was a great cook, and they ate the best of vegan cuisines, smoothies, shakes, sweets, and snacks. The strict vegan lifestyle had done wonders for Ra.

Then one day, I learned Ra was deathly ill with a serious case of colitis, a chronic digestive disease marked by painful inflammation of the colon. He was facing the possibility of being hospitalized and having some of his colon surgically removed. When I finally got ahold of him, he told me the pain had been excruciating and he'd totally lost control of his bowels and even had to wear diapers, it was so unpredictable. On top of that, he'd rapidly lost over thirty pounds— all those fitness gains gone. What was worse, everything Ra was used to eating—all the wide array of plant-based cuisines, and even most leafy greens, veggies, and fruits—were all now irritating to his system. The vegan diet that had given him so much life was now life threatening.

The solution that worked for Ra couldn't have been more surprising to all of us. Grass-fed meats and real butter were some of the only things that would soothe his colon. As he transformed and adapted to what his body was telling him it needed, he would take his own sticks of butter to restaurants, and order things like super rare steaks. Over time and lots of research, he eventually got back to health and then fitness, building himself back into the same physique he had before and then surpassed it. Out of his journey he developed his own "farm to table" fitness philosophy. Ra was now thriving on locally sourced organic meats and butter—the polar opposite of a vegan diet—and I had now witnessed him thrive in both scenarios. I admired my guy's heart and resilience and his ability to change with change.

Waves of Change

My experiences with my own allergy challenges and watching Ra's situation unfold made me realize that determining the "right" diet is a lot more nuanced than the neat little boxes we try to fit in. I was questioning more and more if following a strict vegan diet was still what I needed and wanted.

Afya and I were in the Dominican Republic for a getaway. As we relaxed on the beach at a beautiful resort, staring out at the turquoise Caribbean waters, I heard that intuition voice again.

"I think you should eat fish."

Here I was a decade into my vegan journey, and I hadn't been craving meat or any of the other things I'd left behind. But the nudge of my intuitive voice was compelling, so I mentioned it to Afya.

We were seated at a candlelit table on the beach.

I asked, "Babe, should I eat fish? What if I ate fish?"

She said, "I think you should listen to your body," to my surprise. "The body is wise, and it will ask for what it needs. Then it's up to you to listen or not."

Even though Afya was a longtime vegan health counselor and nutritionist, she was nonjudgmental about me questioning the diet for my body and she was supportive and encouraging.

So, right in that very moment, I decided to order grilled salmon steak and see how it felt—see how *I* felt.

There was a team of beachside chefs cooking up everything fresh on the spot, and man, I ain't gonna lie: that salmon was outstanding. And I didn't experience any funny feelings in my stomach or have a bad reaction. I hadn't eaten fish or any other meat in over ten years. For the rest of our getaway trip, I ordered the same thing and I felt great with no issues. Since that trip back from DR, I've incorporated fish back into my diet. After discovering tree nuts were a no-no for me and that those "wheat meat" substitutes weren't working for me either, I reasoned that fish would be a good source of protein to fill those nutritional gaps. That said, I'm careful to always choose wild-caught fish with the lowest mercury ratings—salmon, cod, and sometimes halibut based on Afya's professional suggestions. The body can and does get rid of mercury over time.

But even so, I'm still somewhat weary about overdoing it because mercury rates are rising daily due to climate change and overfishing. Consuming high levels of mercury over time can be damaging to your kidneys or even lead to nerve issues. So, it's something to be mindful of for sure. The most dangerous type of mercury in fish is called methylmercury. It mainly comes from mercury that exists naturally in ocean sediment and is transformed into methylmercury by micro-organisms. This mercury is absorbed by the tissues of fish through their gills as they swim and through their digestive tracts as they feed. While I personally feel comfortable eating fish to a degree, I'm paying attention to my own body, as you should if you eat fish, to make sure you're not overdoing it. And hey, if you avoid it altogether for any reason, that's an even surer safeguard. Listen to your gut.

I respect the ethical vegan's reasons for not eating meat altogether. I still very much agree with and support the cause to end the unnecessary suffering and slaughter of factory-farm animals, particularly by the fast-food industry. But in full transparency here, I had never gone vegan based on the staunch ethical reasons that many vegans believe in—it was a health choice for me from day one. I have realized that I don't have a moral dilemma with eating fish. I believe, like many indigenous cultures, that there is a natural balance in the equation of life and as a part of nature; just like a bear or a shark does, for me eating fish feels natural. And it sits right with my moral compass.

Coming to this realization after ten years of being a strict vegan, it took me a while to fully settle into accepting that change within myself without worrying about being judged by others as a quitter who turned their back on a lifestyle I was committed to for so long. I'm the type of person that commits to something and then I'm all in, so when things change, I too sometimes question my own values. Was I a quitter? Did I give up on my commitments?

The truth is yes and no. Yes, eating fish is not vegan, so it is what it is; but at the same time, it's not so cut-and-dried, black and white for me. I still do very much advocate for a plant-forward lifestyle. I've experienced countless benefits from maintaining a plant-based lifestyle. I just came to realize that my body was asking for something that didn't fit into the specific ideological box of *vegan* anymore.

And so, I listened to my gut.

BOILED PEANUTS & BOXING

Two peas to a pod.

My pops rarely—and I mean rarely—cooked when I was growing up. My mom made all the magical meals happen in our household. But when Pops did get in the kitchen, it was super special. He would make one of only two things. It was either what Pops referred to as "Cau Pa," a quick stir-fried rice dish with scrambled eggs, sausage, and fresh scallions that he learned to make in Thailand while stationed there in the military, or his other specialty: boiled peanuts.

What you know 'bout boiled peanuts?

Unlike tree nuts, peanuts are related to peas and other legumes. They grow on low green vines, and after they're pollinated, their flower stems turn and burrow down into the ground where they "fruit" into podlike shells. Fresh harvested "green" peanuts go bad fast because of their high moisture, so you have to cook them within a few days of harvesting them out of the ground.

This salty Southern tradition, nicknamed "the caviar of the south," was passed down in our family: from my pops, who learned it from his parents, who in turn learned it from their parents. Papa Luke, my great grandfather, farmed peanuts (among many other things). Back in the day, us kids would help Papa Luke harvest them from the field with rakes, shaking the dirt off the roots and the peanut pods, plucking them from the vine, and filling up wooden barrels with them.

Some of my fondest memories of spending time with my dad are eating boiled peanuts while watching boxing.

In the pitch-dark living room with only the flickering light from the TV, Pops would be sprawled out on the couch shirtless with shorts on, reaching into a bowl full of steaming hot peanuts and grabbing a handful, cracking them open with his teeth, slurping the salty brine from the shells, and nibbling away, while I sat next to him on the floor, enjoying sharing the salty snack, tossing my shells into a plastic bag, mesmerized by the boxing action on-screen: Hagler, Hearns, Holmes, Spinks, Durán, Chávez, Sugar Ray—we watched some classic battles together. Those moments are still so special to me because as life happened and things took a turn for the worse during the eighties and early nineties with the crack epidemic, those special bonding moments were fewer and further between.

I've kept the tradition alive, and when I'm watching boxing and eating boiled peanuts with my sons these days, it always reminds me of the good times I had with my dad. I cherish those memories and strive to keep the tradition going.

COOK UP! POPS'S FIGHT NIGHT PEANUTS

I don't eat oysters, but when I'm eating boiled peanuts, I can imagine it might be something similar to the satisfaction that some people get from eating raw oysters. I love to savor the salty brine inside the shell and scoop out the soft, savory peanut pearls.

But to keep it real, traditionally they are definitely very salty. Pops taught me that you can control how much or how little salt is absorbed in the peanuts by how long you let them sit in the brine. "The longer they sit, the saltier they get." So, you can adjust according to your preference or health concerns. When I make 'em now, I use sea salt instead of the old-school table salt Pops used.

Prep time: 5 minutes (bring to a boil)	Cook time: Boil for about an hour until tender	Makes 8–10 1-cup servings

3 pounds (or so) *fresh green* peanuts in the shells (not dry peanuts, get the fresh green ones)

1 gallon (or so) filtered water or fresh spring or well water

½ cup (or so) sea salt

Wash the peanuts well: Fill a sink or large pot with water, add the peanuts, and stir to remove any dirt. Pour off the dirty water and repeat until the water runs clean.

In a large pot, combine the peanuts with water to cover by 2 inches (about a gallon, more or less depending on the size of your pot). Then add salt (about ½ cup for every gallon of water). This isn't an exact science. Each batch of peanuts is slightly different in moisture content, so how much salt you need will vary. The best

The Four Dimensions

I have my own little theory that I believe speaks to how we go through stages of discovering the truth of ourselves, finding our paths and purposes, and how it all aligns in the grand plan of life.

We go through four dimensions or waves of change as we evolve and grow: from DRAMA→ to DOGMA→ to DHARMA→ to TAO.

DRAMA. The Drama stage, as it sounds, goes in a cycle, from conflict to climax to conflict, back and forth. At this phase, we are just reacting to the conditions we find ourselves in, bumping our heads all thing to do is to taste the brine—you want it to be as salty as you want your boiled peanuts to turn out.

Stir the salt and peanuts and bring to a boil. Lower the flame to medium and put a lid on the pot. Cook for 2 hours, then check to see if they are tender enough for your liking. If not, continue to boil for up to an additional 2 hours. The peanuts' freshness and moisture content determine how long they need to be boiled— keep checking and tasting. Remember: "The longer they sit, the saltier they get."

Drain the peanuts in a colander and transfer to a storage container. They keep well in the fridge for 3 or 4 days.

Now find some classic boxing to watch, like the Hagler vs Hearns trilogy, and enjoy!

Note: The dryer the peanuts are, the more they will float in the water. If this happens, you can place a plate on top of the peanuts to press them down into the pot beneath the water level. Once the peanuts start soaking up the brine, they'll sink, and you can remove the plate.

along the way and doing the best we can with the consciousness we have at that level. We are playing the role we feel we are assigned and supposed to play. And that role is playing out over and over in patterns and cycles of dysfunctional behavior—kept going by the limited perception and perspective of the drama and conflict we are perceiving and experiencing. We are not actors in our own story, we are just reacting to the story we have bought into about ourselves.

DOGMA. To break the drama cycle we look for a dogma, a set of rigid ideas and beliefs to justify and defend what we think, believe, and do, and to help us navigate in the world and feel correct and safe. It's a false guarantee that we give ourselves whatever we want to believe and the dogma that we choose becomes the gospel that we view the world through. Everything that agrees with our dogma is good and right and true and anything that doesn't is bad and wrong and false. This is a powerful but stubborn and limited phase; of course, no one way of seeing things is always right or effective or appropriate in all situations. As the ancient Egyptian proverb reminds us, "Every man is rich in excuses to safeguard his prejudices, his instincts, and his opinions." Once we experience enough scenarios that teach us the limitations of our dogma, we have an opportunity to either evolve our thinking beyond the dogmatic box we've chosen for ourselves, or remain in denial and keep repeating the cycle of dogmatic drama and suffering the consequences of being too rigid and too stubborn for our own good. If we choose to open ourselves up, there's an opportunity to step into our authentic path: Dharma.

DHARMA. Dharma is a Sanskrit term that essentially means truth; your particular authentic path that aligns with your unique makeup. Awakening to your dharma marks when you have found your groove and the flow of your life becomes more effortless. It's not that challenges don't arise, but when you're walking in dharma, you see how the challenges help your path unfold. Instead of resisting change, you see it as a guide to follow. Instead of forcing things, you have found a grace in being that feels as if your life is unfolding perfectly as it should. Resistance and struggle no longer define your journey; acceptance and gratitude guide your path.

TAO. As we live in the power of our dharma and our own authentic being, we start to realize that the destination was and is the journey itself and vice versa. All the drama and dogmas that marked our struggle have led us to our dharma, and nothing was ever not in alignment after all. You see it all plays its part in the harmony of the bigger picture: the Tao, the natural flow of life.

When we move with the Tao, in the grand scheme of things, there is a deep abiding inner peace and knowing that in the highest sense of things—even in the struggles and challenges—all is well, in all ways, always, because at the end of the day, shit is what is—and that's the way it is.

As I've gone through my drama with gout, and then attached myself to the vegan dogma and slowly realized my own dietary dharma, my Tao of nutrition has evolved to a flow that works really well for me. I've come to realize nutrition is not fixed; it changes. A baby doesn't eat the same way a teenager does. A young athlete will eat differently than an elder. A pregnant woman will eat differently than a woman who isn't pregnant.

Nutrition is about having a personal, balanced, functional, flexible, and fluid diet that provides your body with high-quality sources of energy for its needs at different times in life.

Nutrition is not just the food we eat, it's about all of the nourishment we take in: the shows we watch, the music we listen to, the ideas we internalize, and even the company we keep.

I ask myself power questions like: Is this right for me, today? Does this nourish or does this poison? Will eating this or watching this or even thinking particular thoughts bring imbalance and aggravate issues or will it support harmony to mind, body, and spirit? Am I listening to my gut or my taste buds to decide what's best for me?

That's how I do my holistic dance with nutrition these days.

I'm still plant-forward, but the way I currently eat is particular to my own experiences and theories, so I coined my own term for it. Let's get into it!

CHAPTER 7

Vegaquarian

Water is life.

Of all the healthy habits I've picked up from years of practice and soaking up game from Afya, drinking enough water has been one of the practices I've struggled with the most.

The old-school recommendation was to drink at least eight glasses a day. More modern recommendations say drink half the body weight in ounces per day, factoring in a bit more if you have an active lifestyle. But it's tricky: we don't only lose water when we use the bathroom, work out, or sweat on a hot day; we expel water vapor in our breath when we breathe out, and water passes through our skin any time we're in a dry environment, whether it's a desert-like climate or an air-conditioned hotel room.

As explained in the extensive water-metabolism research presented in the classic book *Your Body's Many Cries for Water*, when you're not drinking enough water for things to function properly, the body will "cry out" in many ways. Many chronic health problems are misdiagnosed and are actually a consequence of dehydration—many illnesses and internal issues are the body's way of signaling that it needs more water. We are living rivers, and just like the natural world, the human body has a water regulation system that prioritizes the most essential functions and parts of our bodies for the water we have available in our systems. Our bodies are more than three-fourths water—some say seven-tenths water, approximately the same ratio of water to land on earth—and so it makes sense that we need lots of water for our bodies and minds to function right. It's essential to every aspect of our lives.

Drinking adequate amounts of water boosts energy, strengthens the immune system, and nourishes the skin. It's definitely a great conscious habit to develop. But for me, it's been easier said than done. As much as I've tried to stay on top of it, drinking the recommended daily allowance of water has always taken a huge effort for me and it's an area where I often fall short.

It's also worth noting that it's possible to overdo it by drinking too much water—just like anything else! Mindlessly chugging away in an effort to overcompensate can throw off the normal balance of salts (electrolytes) in the body. Contrary to popular belief, all salt is not to be avoided—we need trace amounts of salt for everything from muscle movement to brain functioning.

In traditional Chinese medicine, the health of the kidney organ system plays a key role in the body's ability to absorb hydration at the cellular level. It's not just about drinking the water. When we are under lots of stress, or we drink too much coffee or alcohol, it negatively impacts the kidneys and that interferes with the body's ability to be properly hydrated among a host of other issues. A benefit of not drinking alcohol or coffee at all (or at least not excessively) and using tools like meditation and other ways to relax is that these practices support hydration by minimizing stress.

So, with all that in mind, being effective and efficient with my hydration game has become a central part of my overall nutrition goals. Over the years, I've had to get more innovative and strategic to make sure I'm getting enough water.

Nutrition is a complex science and I definitely don't consider myself an expert on the subject by any means. But as a student of nutrition in my own life, and in consideration of my particular needs and preferences after years of real-life experimentation, research, and soaking up plenty game from Afya and her insights as a professional nutritionist, currently I'm enjoying a hydration-centered approach to my nutrition that embodies many of the jewels I've picked up along the way.

I call it *vegaquarian*. It breaks down like this: "Vega" represents the entire spectrum of the edible plant kingdom including fermented probiotic-rich plant foods. "Aquarian" represents a distinct emphasis on hydration through select water-rich fruits and veggies, intentional use of water-based cooking methods, and incorporating select fish and seaweeds. Like veganism, no eggs, milk, cheese, or other animal products (except fish) are consumed. So, veggie + aquarian = vegaquarian or VQ for short, which describes my current practice of eating a plant-forward, pescatarian-friendly diet with an emphasis on hydration and digestion.

The approach involves:

- Prioritizing water-rich fruits and veggies
- Including water-based foods like certain fish, seaweeds, and algae
- The intentional use of water-based cooking methods
- The inclusion of fermented and probiotic-rich foods
- Drinking adequate water and hydrating beverages

AWAKEN YOUR SOLE

There is an electrolyte-dense healing brine water remedy called *sole* (pronounced so-lay)—very similar to the word *soul*, no doubt—that is saturated with pink Himalayan salt to mimic the healing salt-to-water ratio of the ocean, which is also the same salt-to-water ratio of our cellular makeup, as well as the same salt-to-water ratio of the embryonic fluid that a baby develops during pregnancy.

Electrolytes are essential for life, assisting the kidneys in eliminating wastes and toxins. They carry a charge which ionizes when dissolved in water. When the water and salt are mixed together, the negative ions of the water molecules combine with the positive ions of salt and vice versa. This way they are electrically charged. The minerals in this drink can be easily absorbed by the body, helping maintain the fluid balance by sending signals from one cell to another.

The benefits of drinking sole are many, but of course if you have high blood pressure or hypertension or any other condition that could possibly make drinking sole unsafe or unwise for you, don't play yourself and have a damn heart attack with this shit—ask your trusted physician what's your best move. If you try it, and experience an immediate negative reaction, stop immediately.

In general, if you have no other health issues that would require you to not do this, here are some of its awesome benefits:

1. BOOSTS YOUR ENERGY: Sole water contains readily bioavailable electrolytes needed to help enhance and sustain your energy at the cellular level. Drinking plain water is great, but some of the essential minerals are flushed out when we do so; as you increase your regular water intake, sole is a good additional supplement as it helps replenish those minerals that may be depleted from your water intake, sweat, and other losses of electrolytes.

2. GET MORE NUTRIENTS IN: Himalayan salt is rich in eighty-four trace minerals and drinking it in the form of sole water makes these minerals and certain other important vitamins more bioavailable and easier to absorb by the body.

3. A WIN FOR YOUR SKIN: Certain minerals in Himalayan salt help fight many skin problems. Among many other benefits, zinc, iodine, chromium, and sulfur have multiple benefits, many related to healthy skin, from repairing tissues to preventing acne and resolving skin infections.

4. PEACE AND CALM: Sole water calms the entire nervous system and helps you relax. The salt minerals help reduce stress hormones which carries the benefit of better sleep and a more peaceful state of mind in general.

5. DOPE FOR DIGESTION: Himalayan salt stimulates metabolism (the breaking down of food for energy) and also assists the intestinal tract and the liver in doing their digestive functions.

COOK UP! SOLE VEGAQUARIAN

If you're ready to charge up your hydration and mineral absorption, here's a "sole satisfying" recipe and remedy.

To make the concentrated sole, fill a 32-ounce plastic-lidded glass jar one-fourth with pink Himalayan salt. Add water to the top of the jar. Close the lid, shake vigorously, and let it sit overnight.

In the morning (or 8 hours later), the salt should be fully dissolved in the water. If some remains undissolved, shake again and leave until no more salt is floating in the water. At this time, your sole concentrate is ready. Do not drink the concentrated solution.

Add 1 teaspoon sole concentrate for every 32 ounces drinking water. Replenish as needed throughout the day. Try it for 3 days and see how you feel.

The Rainforest Connection

I've been an urban city dweller for many years of my life, but I'm still a country boy at heart. I find so much inspiration in the natural world. My VQ concept draws inspiration from the model of a thriving rainforest ecosystem.

There is an ancient ecological concept that in modern times has been called the *Gaia hypothesis;* this is the theory that the Earth is a living, self-regulating being that proactively creates the conditions to support life. The rich and complex activities of the rainforest offer convincing evidence for that case.

Rainforest 101

There are two types of rainforests—temperate and tropical.

Temperate rainforests are much lower in temperature than tropical rainforests and they tend to be farther from the equator, in places like Australia, New Zealand, Chile, and the UK, as well as certain areas of North America.

Tropical rainforests, on the other hand, are very hot and thrive near the equator. Many get an inch or more of rain every day of the year. The largest tropical rainforest in the world is the Amazon, which spans over more than two and a half million square miles of South America. Central America, Asia, and Australia also have tropical rainforests.

Rainforests play a vital role in keeping our planet healthy and their functioning is critically important for our well-being. They've been called "the lungs of the planet" because of the massive amounts of carbon dioxide they absorb, which helps to stabilize the Earth's climate.

Rainforests also help produce massive amounts of nourishing rainfall all around the planet and it's been estimated that more than a quarter of all medicines originate from their tropical forest plants.

Rainforests are the most essential, abundant, biodiverse, resilient ecosystems we have on Earth. Rainforests are the embodiment of a rich, balanced, thriving, sustainable way of life. They are literally real-life paradises.

Biomimicry (Bi·o·mim·ic·ry) is a term used to describe the human-designed systems that are inspired by the wisdom of nature. It refers to relying on the models, systems, and elements of nature for the purpose of providing solutions for our complex human needs.

It's my theory that the fundamental characteristics of a thriving rainforest present us with a master guide for nutrition and hydration, and by *"bio-mimic-ing"* the rainforest's characteristic principles in our approach to nutrition we can embody the same kind of sustainable vitality that rainforests have.

Rainforests—The Four Nutritional Elements

A thriving rainforest has four key elements: **high rainfall, intense sunlight, immense biodiversity,** and **highly absorptive soil.** These elements of the rainforest ecosystem are the combined key factors that drive and sustain the rainforest's vitality.

Let's unpack how each piece fits into vegaquarian nutrition.

High Rainfall

As the name suggests, rainforests play a huge role in the water cycle by creating, in some places, over 75 percent of their own rainfall.

VQ applies the principle of high rainfall by putting focus on hydration—and lots of it. One way this is implemented is by striving to drink half the body's weight in ounces daily. Another is prioritizing whole foods that have a naturally high water content. And still another way we "bio·mimic" the high rainfall element is by incorporating water-based cooking methods like steaming, boiling, poaching, and blanching.

Intense Sunlight

The sun obviously plays a profound role in the rainforest. The 90-degree angle of sunlight that hits the equator year-round provides plants with abundant solar energy for photosynthesis, and rainforest trees and plants excel at converting that light into a cornucopia of diverse, chlorophyll-rich and nutrient-dense fruits and vegetables that sustain the massive array of animals, insects, and microorganisms that live and thrive there.

In one way or another, we all get our energy from the sun—its solar power is transformed and stored as energy in the plants and animals we eat. The vegaquarian application of the intense sunlight element in practice is achieved by choosing energizing, nutrient-dense foods, including a bountiful variety of colorful, organic whole foods; fresh fruits; veggies; herbs; nuts and seeds; mushrooms; herbal teas; wild-caught, low mercury–rated fish like salmon, halibut, and cod; as well as seaweeds, kelp, and edible algae.

This principle is also applied by making sure to include plenty of fruits and vegetables in their raw "sun-cooked" state to take advantage of the live enzymes they contain.

Immense Biodiversity

Rainforests only cover about 6 percent of the Earth's land surface but more than 50 percent of all land species in the world live there. That's over half the creatures in the world!

Applying the principle of biodiversity in a vegaquarian practice is all about maintaining a well-rounded, diversified, plant-rich diet full of seasonal variety, making room on our plates and in our kitchens for a full range of seasonal, organic foods as often as possible. It's great when you've finally found favorite foods that work well for you and that you enjoy, but it's equally important to challenge ourselves to try new things in search of a well-rounded cross section of nutrients in the diet throughout the year. Applying the wisdom of biodiversity means intentionally aligning our nutrition strategy with what the planet is naturally yielding at different times of the year in our local environments as much as possible.

Highly Absorptive Soil

The final jewel on the vegaquarian crown is focused on good digestive absorption.

The soil in the rainforest has a unique quality. You would think the soil would be rich because of all the abundant plant life the rainforest supports but the opposite is true. Rainforest soil is actually very poor in terms of holding on to nutrients. All of the rainfall washes away nutrients at a much higher and faster rate than other forests. With all the high humidity from all the rain and intense heat, there is always a thick layer of rapidly decaying plants and animals on top of the soil.

The nutrients from the rotting and fermenting organic matter is relentlessly washed by the heavy rains and absorbed into the growing plants and trees, so the soil doesn't actually get to hold on to nutrients very long. But who knows what's good or bad? This "nutrient-poor soil" is what allows rapid absorption of nutrients by the surrounding trees and plants, and that's why they are able to grow and thrive with the tremendous strength and nutritional potency that they have.

In my VQ model, all this translates as an apt metaphor for good gut health.

For our own nutrient absorption process to work well, we need a healthy gut and a strong digestive system. If our digestion or gut health is not functioning well, we won't absorb nutrients well and that's like finding a gold mine and loading up the bounty, only to realize that you've got a hole in your bag.

"*Biomimicing*" the rich, absorptive principle of rainforest soil in the vegaquarian practice looks like this:

Respecting and incorporating fermented foods: Fermented foods, such as nonpasteurized pickles, sauerkraut, kimchi, kombucha, and one of my favorite Ethiopian staples injera, all contain natural probiotics that are great for the gut and help in optimizing digestion.

Adding and enjoying live foods: Again, raw foods have more live enzymes available than cooked foods, generally speaking, and coupled with the higher water content they contain, they help digestion function more smoothly. Note here: from the perspective of traditional Chinese medicine, our acupuncturist has advised at times to minimize raw fruits and veggies for certain periods when a person has certain digestive challenges or imbalances. So, as with all things, be a good student; don't just accept none of this stuff as a rigid gospel. There are always exceptions. Do the knowledge for what works best for your body.

Absorption pairing: Taking the gut health tips a step further, in addition to cutting out toxic substances, detoxing seasonally, and avoiding foods that irritate my gut or cause allergic reactions, I've also learned to maximize the nutrients in my diet by implementing a practice called absorption pairing. Absorption pairing is yet another creative technique to explore with your nutrition, based on combining, mixing, and matching specific foods that have increased digestive benefits when eaten or "paired" together, promoting maximum absorption of nutrients. If you want to improve absorption pairing, squeeze some lemon juice onto iron-rich foods. The vitamin C in citrus fruits targets and enhances the extraction of iron. And it's not just citrus; other vitamin C–rich foods such as cauliflower, brussels sprouts, chilies, and peppers combine with iron-rich legumes or beets for maximum impact!

Striking nutrient oil: Take, for example, vitamins A, D, E, and K, which are in many vegetables and are all fat-soluble, meaning they require fat to be digested properly. To oversimplify the body's intricate digestive wisdom, mindfully consuming veggies with these vitamins along with healthy fats helps the body absorb these nutrients quickly and efficiently. That might mean using coconut, flaxseed, or olive oil or adding fatty nuts, seeds, and avocados to your meals to enhance the vitamin absorption from your veggie platter.

Water Your Garden

I can't stress enough how important it is to maintain hydration. Here are a few other quick hacks that I've landed on to get more hydration in my days.

First Things First—I don't drink coffee. I start my day with a cup or two of water; this is the best way to keep hydration on my mind for the rest of the day. Coffee is actually very dehydrating—the high caffeine content taxes the kidneys and liver to filter it.

Chlorophyll Sippin'—A squirt of liquid chlorophyll adds a fresh nutritional boost to your water. (Thank Badu for this one!) My boy, Coach NYM, and I have made sipping green gallons a ritual in the lab when we cooking up new music. When we're working on a project for long hours in the studio, we'll each get a gallon of water and add a few droplets of the "green plant blood" and sip on that throughout our sessions. It keeps us hydrated, enhances our nutrient intake, and breaks the monotony of regular water.

Everyday Carry—Keeping a water bottle on deck at all times is a must: in the car, in my bag, on my bedside table. It's always conveniently near and helps me remember to drink my daily quota throughout the day. I keep a copper flask for my everyday water bottle. The oldest recorded medical use of copper comes from an ancient African medical text back in 2200 BC that describes the use of copper to sterilize drinking water and treat wounds for infection. In the thousands-of-years-old Eastern Indian Ayurvedic healing tradition, copper is an extremely important mineral that not only kills bacteria, but can also positively charge water and help bring better balance to mind, body, and spirit. The copper gently seeps into the water and instills it with powerful healing properties. Storing water in copper also extends its "life" and keeps it from going stale. Whatever you use, try to avoid plastic bottles, especially on hot days, since the heat can cause them to leach chemicals into your water supply.

Drinking on the Clock—I've found it helpful to schedule my hydration. Starting in the a.m. when I first wake up, I set my alarm to alert me every three hours to have at least sixteen ounces of water. So that could look like drinking sixteen ounces of water at 9:00 a.m., 12:00 p.m., 3:00 p.m., 6:00 p.m., and 9:00 p.m. That's five intervals of sixteen ounces of water each for a total of eighty ounces, which is about half my body weight. You can adjust the increments for your daily requirements.

Stay Soakin' Up Game—Continuing to research and find good reads on water helps me remain mindful, motivated, and intentional with drinking water and staying hydrated. One of the absolute best books I've ever read on water that I highly recommend is *The Hidden Secrets of Water* by Dr. Paolo Consigli. You've never been so fully entertained and enlightened on the subject of water as you will be reading that joint, trust me! And another deeply profound book on water is *Water & Salt: The Essence of Life* by Dr. Barbara Hendel and Peter Ferreira.

Now, if all this vegaquarian food and drink talk is making you hungry and thirsty, I've got just the thing to bring it all home.

The Broth of Life

The epitome of an example that can embody all the aforementioned vegaquarian principles is—you ready? Drumroll please . . . soup!

Soups are satisfying, energizing, and filling, and the multiple flavors in the broth are rich, layered, and unlimited in how savory and sophisticated they can be. Soup is the perfect vessel to apply all the vegaquarian, rainforest-inspired strategies in one bowl! Here's how soup shapes up as a perfect meal, incorporating all the nutritional elements.

High Rainfall. By definition, broths and soups are usually water based and have high water content, so soups are highly hydrating.

Intense Sunlight & Biodiversity. You can significantly increase the nutrient diversity, quality and quantity, by incorporating any and all veggies, fish, rice, etc., you have on hand into your soup.

Absorption and Digestion. Soup served hot opens up the sweat channels and helps improve blood flow and circulation. The long, slow preparation and low-to-medium-heat cooking process gently breaks down the soup's ingredients, making nutrients more available by the time the first spoonful hits your mouth. Also, because warm soups are gentle on the gastrointestinal system and supportive in hydrating the body's various systems, they are one of the most digestion-friendly meals you can eat.

COOK UP! RAINFOREST SOUP WITH SALMON AND RICE

One of my absolute favorite vegaquarian meals is what I've dubbed rainforest soup. It's rich in flavors from around the world and has become one of my staples, with its hearty, aromatic coconut milk–based broth and medley of both fresh and organic frozen vegetables, herbs, and spices, and a generous squeeze of lemon. I top it with cardamon-infused jasmine or basmati rice and pan-seared, wild-caught salmon, then garnish with crispy nori strips. Soups are medicinal meals and the food equivalent of a warm hug. You can eat off this soup for days if you're just cooking for one, but even if you've got a family of four or more, everyone can enjoy seconds and thirds. Enjoy!

Prep time: 20 minutes   Cook time: 45 minutes   Makes 4 servings

Soup

- 1/4 cup coconut oil
- 2 to 4 tablespoons minced garlic, to taste
- 2 cups water, plus more as needed
- 1 tablespoon nondairy margarine
- 3-4 cardamom pods
- 2 tablespoons sea salt (to taste)
- 2-3 teaspoons black pepper (to taste)
- 2-3 teaspoons onion powder (to taste)
- 2-3 teaspoons garlic powder (to taste)
- 2 teaspoons smoked paprika
- 2-3 teaspoons lemon pepper
- 2 teaspoons garam masala powder
- 5 teaspoons umami mushroom powder (to taste)
- 1-2 (12-ounce) bags frozen mixed vegetable medley (I like the classic mix of carrots, green beans, sweet peas, and corn)
- 1 to 2 (15-ounce cans or bags or carton) chickpeas, drained
- 1 head fresh cauliflower, cut into florets
- 10 to 15 cherry tomatoes, sliced in half
- 1 (13.5-ounce) can organic unsweetened coconut milk
- Juice of 1/2 fresh lemon
- Sprigs of fresh herbs, such as rosemary, thyme, marjoram—even bay leaf (optional)

Salmon

- 4 (6-ounce) wild-caught frozen salmon fillets, skin on, deboned
- 4 teaspoons lemon juice, plus more for seasoning
- 1 teaspoon onion powder
- 1 teaspoon lemon pepper
- 1 teaspoon sea salt
- 1/2 teaspoon black pepper
- 1 tablespoon coconut oil

Rice

- 2 cups jasmine or basmati rice (see Notes)
- About 4 cups water
- I teaspoon nondairy margarine
- 2 or 3 cardamom pods
- I or 2 pinches sea salt
- I teaspoon turmeric (optional)
- Chopped green onions (scallions)
- Crispy nori strips, cut into thin slices like confetti
- Lemon juice
- Pinch red pepper flakes

Make the soup: Heat the coconut oil in a large soup pot over medium-low heat. Add the garlic and sauté for 2 to 4 minutes, until it starts to brown. Add the water, margarine, and all the spices.

As it starts to boil, pour in additional water to fill the pot about three-fourths full. You can always add more water if you find you need it. Add the mixed veggies, chickpeas, cauliflower florets, and cherry tomatoes. Stir in the coconut milk and squeeze in the lemon juice. Taste the broth and add additional seasonings to taste.

Turn the heat to high and bring everything to a boil. Add the fresh herbs—if you wrap a cooking string around the sprigs or put them in a cloth tea pouch, they will be easy to remove.

Reduce the heat to medium-low, cover, and simmer until the cauliflower is tender, 25 to 30 minutes. Keep the pot simmering on low heat and serve hot.

Make the salmon: Meanwhile, season the fillets all over with the lemon juice, onion powder, lemon pepper, salt, and pepper and let marinate while the pan gets hot.

Heat a skillet over medium heat for about 3 minutes. Add the coconut oil and heat until simmering. Add the salmon fillets to the pan, skinned side down, one at a time, pressing down and rubbing each on the bottom of the pan to lightly sear each side and spread the oil around really well. (This helps keep the salmon from sticking.) Cook, flipping the fillets after 3 to 5 minutes, until they're browned how you like them. Salmon is done when it flakes easily with a fork. I like mine super well-done, and I mash the fillets down with a spatula to get that slight crispy texture.

Make the rice: Follow the instructions on the package to cook the rice (it's usually a ratio of 2 cups water to 1 cup rice, but check your package): Bring the water to a boil over high heat. Add the rice, margarine, cardamom, and sea salt. If you want yellow rice, add the turmeric. Stir a few times, and when it is all boiling, reduce the heat to medium and cover with a lid. Cook for about 20 minutes (or according to package instructions), until the water is absorbed and the rice is light and tender. Turn off the heat and keep covered.

Bring it all together: Now your rice is fluffy and ready, your soup is aromatic and steaming, and your salmon is well done, moist, and sizzling hot.

For each serving, ladle soup into a bowl, then add some rice and place a seared salmon fillet on top of the rice. Garnish with green onions and nori strips, then add another squeeze of lemon juice and a pinch of red pepper flakes for a spicy kick. And boom! There you have it. A savory, satisfying, hydrating, nutrient-dense, diverse, digestion-friendly, delicious, and nutritious symphony of rainforest wisdom in your bowl.

Notes: Use fresh springwater or filtered water and all organic ingredients whenever possible.

I prefer jasmine or basmati rice but you should use whatever you prefer: brown rice, millet, quinoa—it's your world. While some folks say it's not necessary to rinse rice, it's good to do so in order to remove dirt, dust, debris, chemicals, and/or bugs that may remain from the harvesting process. Rinsing your rice before you cook it also helps remove excess starch and gives your finished rice a fluffier texture, with individually separated rice kernels instead of a gummy, mushy, sticky texture.

Nutrition Goes beyond Food

Nutrition is more than the fruits, vegetables, grains, nuts, seeds, herbs, fish, and so forth that we consume. The goal of nutrition is a vital, energized life, and all of the energy, experiences, and information we bring into our lives on physical, mental, and spiritual levels are a part of our "nutritional" practice.

What We Nourish Will Flourish

When we're well hydrated and nourished with a variety of nutrients, we can thrive holistically. The vegaquarian framework is where I landed through exploration and experimentation with what works for me, and I think it can provide many benefits for you, too. So, make it yours. Add elements from my vegaquarian approach to your diet and customize it to your own lifestyle, preferences, and needs. VQ is not meant to be a stand-alone diet or a set of hard-and-fast rules to eat by; it's a simple way to add more hydration and nourishment to accent and supplement your otherwise healthy intake of proteins, fats, carbs, vitamins, and minerals. Make sure you check with your doctor, nutritionist, or trusted health-care provider to make sure VQ is a good fit for your particular needs. Everybody is different. Listen to your gut. What we nourish will flourish.

OUR DIET NEEDS TO BE MORE PLANT BASED,
MORE GREENS, MORE WATER, BECAUSE OUR
BODIES ARE LIKE PLANTS.

—PRODIGY, OF MOBB DEEP (RIP)

CHAPTER 8

Kitchen Kung Fu

You can only know what you are really consuming when you make it yourself.

Nutrition is an action sport. And unless you've got a personal chef and a live-in maid on call, healthier living requires you to get busy in the kitchen. That's just the facts, fam. Some folks are already accustomed to cooking and kitchen work so making the shift to cooking healthier doesn't require that much of a learning curve—they already have basic kitchen skills and might just need to make better nutritional choices with the ingredients they chef up. But if you're just starting out on the path of taking your health more seriously, you start to realize right away that you can't be lazy about being healthy.

Learning to Cook

This is a key skill for maintaining a healthy lifestyle. If you don't cook or have a personal chef on your payroll to cook whatever you ask them to cook, your nutrition is pretty much at the mercy of what someone else cooks or what you can afford to buy from restaurants. Relying on restaurants and delivery gets costly, too.

Now, I love going out to restaurants, just like anybody does. It's so convenient and satisfying to sit down at a nice place and explore the menu, make your selection, and just sit back and enjoy the delicious hard work of the chefs or cooks in the back. No food to prepare, no dishes to do, just eat, enjoy, and relax. I mean that's what we pay for at restaurants right? We should enjoy it.

But do we really know what's in what we are eating? How much salt is in that soup? Is the vegetable oil soybean or canola or olive? Do you really know how much added sugar is in that sauce? Is your overworked and underpaid server really that knowledgeable and sensitive to your food-allergy concerns? What about food coloring or additives or preservatives? Is the fish wild caught or farm raised? Are the veggies organic or grown in pesticides? Is this rice fresh or several days old and reheated? Did they heat this hot water for tea in a microwave?

Cooking for ourselves at home cuts out the guessing games. When you're at the helm, you can make sure nothing you're allergic to or don't wanna eat goes into your pot, pan, plate, or mouth.

Cooking for yourself makes you more aware of the quality of the ingredients in what you're eating. And it makes you feel more self-reliant and responsible for your own nourishment and well-being.

I also find that cooking helps me be more mindful of what I'm eating when I'm eating. When you've put your heart and mind into making a meal from scratch, you tend to pay attention to every bite and savor your food more when you're eating it. This simple act of mindfulness also helps us recognize when we've had enough and when we listen to our gut and don't overdo it, that supports better digestion.

You can best believe that one of the most important things you can do to start eating healthier is to start cooking your own food. Ordering takeout every once in a white ain't gonna kill you on the spot, but after a while, a steady stream of fast food and microwave meals lowers our vitality, and we settle into a low vibrational pattern of eating that saps our energy and undermines our health. Living off

Styrofoam staples just out of convenience, because we don't feel like cooking or don't wanna do dishes, is an unhealthy habit in and of itself.

Microwaving might be super convenient, but at what cost to our long-term health? Taking the time to put love and care into a home-cooked meal compared to microwaving is like comparing passionate lovemaking to a meaningless moment of masturbation. One is quicker but—well, you get the point. And hey, no judgment—sometimes we gotta do what we gotta do!

Seriously, your relationship with your kitchen and ingredients is a powerful one. It's literally a matter of life and death. If disease begins in the colon, our nutritional health is cultivated in the kitchen.

Bringing the healthy attitude of respect to your kitchen as a creative space for nourishment makes a world of difference.

In *The Karate Kid*, when Daniel-san eventually realized that the repetitive "wax on, wax off" work he had to do to bring the shine back to an old jalopy actually revealed deeper meaning, application, and purpose—as well as a classic car hiding in plain sight—I've discovered over the years that the kitchen is a powerful place not only to practice healthy cooking, but it's also a dojo of powerful life lessons waiting to be realized.

Culinary Kung Fu

In the Western world, "kung fu" is often used to describe Chinese martial arts, but that's not the full meaning. The more accurate term for Chinese martial arts is *wushu*. The real meaning of kung fu is *skill*—any study, learning, or practice that requires patience, energy, and time to develop. It's the principle of sincere effort—devotion, discipline, and dedication applied to any practice or craft. Kung fu can be expressed in many aspects of life; it's that good old "what you put in is what you get out" work ethic in any and everything we do.

That's where kitchen kung fu kicks in.

I'm no Iron Chef by any means, but being married to an award-winning plant-based cookbook author and nutritionist for many moons, plus raising two little ninjas that like to eat—often—I've picked up a few hacks that make my life easier in the kitchen.

Here are four fundamental techniques and timeless time-saving tips to kick-start your kitchen kung fu:

1. **RESPECT YOUR DOJO: Just as kung fu isn't limited to martial arts, a dojo isn't simply a space where martial arts are practiced.** A dojo is any place of sincere practice, so in this sense, the kitchen also is a dojo—the heart of a healthy lifestyle practice. So, while some folks function just fine in messy kitchens, I'm just not one of those folks. I've got to work clean. It's a mental dojo thing for me. Dojos are treated with reverence and respect; dojos are kept orderly and clean. Maintain your kitchen space with the same level of respect and reverence as you would a dojo. It's a mindset, and no matter if it's the kitchen, training hall, or anywhere else, your mind is the innermost dojo.

2. **SIMPLIFY: Home cooking don't have to be all complex and difficult.** Of course, there are levels to the culinary arts, but healthy cooking can actually be pretty easy. Following a recipe in a cookbook is just like following a to-do list. Maybe you start with making one meal a week. Or make enough to eat on for multiple days in the week. Then build up your go-to recipes as you go. Grilling, blending, boiling, broiling, chopping, slicing, sautéing, baking, or lightly stir frying—none of those methods are rocket science. You can be inspired by Top Chefs but you ain't gotta try and top them to eat well. You don't need to do too much. You don't necessarily have to be putting the ingredients through all

kinds of extra processing: the simplest foods be the healthiest foods, and keeping your food preparation methods simple makes healthy cooking pretty easy—and other than some overnight soaking and marination here and there, pretty fast, too.

3. **MISE EN PLACE / KITCHEN KATA: In karate practice, a kata is a simple form or movement that is repeated routinely to create muscle memory until the action becomes second nature.** The French culinary phrase *mise en place* points to the same thing; inspired by French military routines, the system is often used in busy restaurants to organize ingredients and establish an efficient workflow for the kitchen crew. Mise en place means "everything in its right place," and just like a series of kata in the kitchen, the systems and routines we set up for efficiency and cleanliness keep things in order and running smoothly.

    Again, simplicity is the goal. The whole idea is to create and maintain a realistic system of where things go, how and when they're used, and how your tools—pots, pans, appliances, knife sets, and utensils—are organized in ways and spaces that make sense for your smoothest flow. When you're cheffing up a meal, or making a smoothie, whipping up some fresh guac, or simply putting away a grocery-store haul, lean into your system and let it work for you. Put groceries away as soon as you walk in the door. Return ingredients to their organized place right when you're done with them. And of course, remember ABC: always be cleaning—that applies to everything from wiping down surfaces as you go to washing the dishes in the sink as they accumulate. I don't know about you, but keeping things in order supports my mental health. So, I make sure to replace the messiness with mise en place.

4. **WORKING CLEAN: Cooking and cleaning the kitchen are sometimes under-acknowledged as necessary**

skills of healthy living. A steady cycle of cooking breakfast, lunch, and dinner—and then washing and putting away the dishes that accumulate—can seem like a grind day in and day out, and it may be a deterrent for people who don't wanna put in that work. But if we look at it maturely, we know that nourishing ourselves and cleaning up after ourselves are aspects of self-care and self-reliance that are highly important and build character in our lives. The key is keeping things simple, manageable, and clean as you go so it doesn't become overwhelming. It's better to tackle kitchen duties proactively than to just let mess and clutter pile up and violate your home sanctuary. I always remind myself to be grateful that I even have food to eat and a kitchen to clean up.

COOK UP! THE GREATEST GUACAMOLE

I'm the guac maker of the family and I'm damn proud of it! This is my secret recipe. I'm only sharing it with you 'cause we are cool like that and I feel like you will respect the tradition with your life. Got that? Judging by how quickly it disappears out of the bowl once I tell the family it's ready, it's pretty delicious, if I do say so myself. Making great guacamole is all about the quality of the ingredients. Try to use fresh and organic ingredients if you can. You'll need a medium bowl and something to mash the guac with, or if you have a stone bowl and a mortar and pestle, even better.

Prep time: 10 minutes   Makes 4 servings

3 or 4 ripe but firm black Hass avocados, pitted and peeled	1/2 cup of minced fresh cilantro
1/2 yellow onion, diced	Juice of 1/2 lime
1 tomato	Sea salt to taste, I like about 1/4 teaspoon or so

In a medium bowl, combine the avocado, onion, tomato, cilantro, lime juice, and salt. Mash together until blended; it should be creamy but still chunky. Serve with organic blue chips, sliced or baby carrots, or use in sandwiches. Enjoy the greatness!

Tools of the Trade

Every healthy kitchen needs certain things to work. Here's a brief list of essential appliances and tools in our kitchen.

WATER FILTER: The quality—or the toxicity—of public water systems varies from community to community. Just ask the folks in Flint, Michigan: the city's contaminated water led to reports of rashes, itchy skin, and hair loss before a state-appointed commission declared the lack of governmental response to be the result of systemic racism. No shit! The point is, just as you keep your guard up with any martial art, kitchen kung fu is no different. Leave nothing to chance. We use filtered water for all our cooking, tea brewing... even ice making! Buying bottled water gets pricey over time and it ain't the most environmentally friendly choice either, so consider investing in a high-quality water filter attached to your kitchen faucet—or a sleek stainless-steel system for your countertop—and save some of that bottled water money to buy my albums!

QUALITY OVER QUANTITY: Speaking from experience, investing in cookware will elevate your kitchen kung fu by getting you motivated to make magic happen with quality tools. Take time to assemble your dojo with different-size stockpots, baking pans, and skillets. Sometimes it's easiest to grab a basic set of these when they're on sale, but keep your eyes peeled for vintage finds like cast-iron skillets that acquire character over time, getting blacker and stronger every time they're put in the fire.

ELECTRIC KETTLE: In the past, we used to use the stovetop to boil water, but then we discovered electric kettles. These convection devices save time by getting water hot in seconds, and they save energy as well—some models are 50 percent more efficient than stovetops when it comes to boiling water. Not only do we use that water for tea, we also use it when making spaghetti noodles, soups, or boiled peanuts. If you absolutely have to have a microwave where you live, try to use it as little as possible.

STOVETOP GRILL PAN / GRIDDLE: When blazing veggies outdoors ain't an option, grill pans are designed to be used on the stovetop or in the oven. Their deep ridges mimic a standard grill rack and go a long way toward bringing through that backyard taste and texture. Ours is made of cast iron to handle high heat, but they come in a range of styles from nonstick to electric.

FOOD PROCESSOR: Where a blender, well, blends...a food processor basically chops up ingredients to varying degrees in a matter of seconds—cutting up veggies for a recipe or chopping nuts down to make your own homemade nut butters. The uses are endless.

BLENDER: Can't make your daily smoothie without a blender. Nuff said. In our kitchen, we make so many smoothies we use an industrial-strength Vitamix!

GLASS STORAGE CONTAINERS: Another quality move—unlike plastic, glass doesn't stain, peel, or—most importantly—take on the taste or odor of the food stored in them. Ideal for airtight sealing of leftovers or fresh prepped cuts at room temperature, in the refrigerator, or in the freezer, these come in a range of sizes from a single cup to several quarts.

KNIFE TRAINING / KNOW YOUR KNIFE: Owning a quality chef's knife and getting up on basic knife technique will speed up recipe prep time (and reduce the risk of injury). Online tutorials are a good place to start learning, but also check for intro classes at cooking supply shops and even continuing ed programs. In the meantime, get to work on practicing basic movements like chopping (cutting into uniform chunks), dicing (smaller chunks), mincing (tiny pieces), and slicing vegetables (julienne) and herbs (chiffonade). Learn and practice simple knife skills, and your prep will not only be smoother, it will be safer. Pay close attention at all times when handling knives; hold the knife firmly by the handle, cut away from—not toward—the body, and put away knives securely when not in use. And be extra careful with fruits with big pits like mangos and avocados!

MASTER YOUR GROCERY RUNS: It sucks being in the middle of cheffing up greatness only to discover you're out of a key ingredient. Keep a master grocery list at a designated spot in the kitchen or as a shareable note in your phone to jot down ingredients and supplies as they run out. Consider all the food groups as well as your usual favorites or specific recipe ingredients so instead of relying on memory, you can refer to the list when you're active at the grocery store. Encourage others in your household to contribute to the list, too.

BULK COOKING: It takes more or less the same amount of time to make one cup of rice as it does a whole pot. Cooking in bulk batches saves time down the road, so instead of making a bowl for one meal, why not make enough rice for the week? It will save you time later.

LESS IS MORE: Let's be real. Do you really need seventeen bowls, thirty-two plates, and forty-five spoons? The more dishes you have, the more dishes you have to wash and put away. Consider limiting dishes to one or two for every person in your household, and instead of reaching for a clean plate because the sink is piled high with dirty ones...how about just wash the dishes in the sink? It's like that old idea that the more time you give yourself to do something, the more time it will take—fewer dishes to wash means more time for other things you enjoy!

I have moments of insight when I'm doing mundane tasks like washing dishes. Just recently, I left a pot of peanuts too long on the stove—the inside of that joker was burnt black with no hope of saving it. I tried scrubbing it but no dice. After some thought, I decided to leave it soaking in some hot soapy water. When I returned, I got busy scrubbing it with circular motions, and boom! That stubborn layer of burnt peanuts started to give way. It took a forearm workout but after a while the whole pot was clean as new.

It dawned on me that life is like this. In the face of a challenge, sometimes we need to be like that burnt pot soaking in water, just sitting and allowing time to pass for the possibilities in the situation to loosen up. It may still take some elbow grease, but in the end, we'll start to see our efforts have a positive effect. That's the wisdom of patience balanced with effort. Being present in our kitchen katas— or any activities for that matter—allows opportunities to experience these mundane moments mindfully and pick up gems in the process. We don't have to just do the dishes—we can Tao the dishes.

Food is fun, culture, and life—enjoy it! You absolutely can make and enjoy delicious, nutritious meals at home and fall in love with the process along the way. You ain't gotta be a Michelin-star chef, but as you grow in knowledge, wisdom, and understanding about what it means to take responsibility for your own healthy nutrition, basic kitchen skills come in handy. A household with hungry kids running around makes this even more essential. Cooking can be time consuming, but with some basic efficiency techniques and a mature outlook, that kitchen kung fu will support your healthy choices with irreplaceable life skills. And you'll be the sensei of your stovetop in no time.

OUS!

FIND YOUR FITNESS

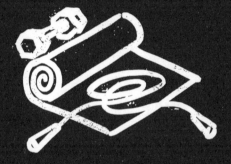

CHAPTER 9

Walk like a Warrior

You never know how strong you are until being strong
is the only choice you have.

—*Bob Marley*

The Inuit people have a beautiful practice called the anger walk. If a tribe member gets angry, they are given a stick and sent to walk in a straight line out into the arctic landscape. They have to keep walking until they feel their anger has been resolved. Then, the tribe member pitches their anger stick into the ice, marking the length and strength of the rage. And then they can come back. The real magic in this is that they actually have to walk twice as far as they thought (there and back), so by the time they're all the way back, they've had twice the time to thaw out and are in a much better state of mind.

If I lived there, I could imagine my country ass saying, "I was past-the-seals mad at that girl!" or, "This fool had me beyond-the-polar-bears pissed!"

But seriously, that's a beautiful tradition, right? Walking is that powerful.

New York City is one of the best cities for walking in the world and I loved going on long walks when I lived there. When my ankle had completely healed from gout and all the swelling and pain was gone, I had a whole new level of energy at my disposal. I ain't wanna sit still. All that clean, green eating was giving me life. Just to be able to walk on my own two down the street, pain free, felt like an occasion for celebration.

Until I was back on my feet, I hadn't realized how much I missed my weekend strolls along the tree-lined brownstones of Brooklyn or midday hikes in the hustle and bustle of Manhattan. Some days, I've walked all the way from Harlem down to the Lower East Side. There's so much to see, so much culture to spark you. Art. Fashion. Style. Vinyl. Books. Colorful graffiti on the buildings and trains. It's a gritty, creative landscape with inspiration everywhere. When you're walking in NY, it feels like you don't even get tired 'cause you're constantly being charged up by all the sights and scenes of the city. As the saying goes, health is wealth, and for me, walking with a recently healed leg through New York City again made me feel like a million bucks!

Walking is such an underrated exercise. It's easy to do, it costs nothing, there's no real risk of injury, and it's great for the heart. When we get out and walk, we're burning calories, stimulating circulation, and increasing muscle tone in our legs. It's also an opportunity to unplug for a while, slow down, and notice things more both in our environments and in ourselves. After healing my leg and getting back on my feet in full stride, walking was no longer just walking; every step was a personal victory lap.

One day I was walking from the 'Stuy back to Crown Heights and I happened to look up and notice a sign that I'd probably passed a zillion times before but never saw:

WORLD FITNESS CENTER

I thought, what's that?

I went up the one flight of stairs on the side of the concrete building, opened the framed glass door, and walked inside to check it out.

The layout was clean: hardwood floors, giant mirrors across the back wall, standard exercise equipment like bikes, hand weights, and male and female changing rooms. It was a nice space. The brother working there, who I later learned was the owner, was a muscular, dark-skinned man with a thick Caribbean accent and an open-face gold-tooth crown. He was making his rounds with keys on his waist, wiping and cleaning while a few folks scattered around and got their workout in. I'd satisfied my curiosity and I was making my way to the exit when I picked up a flyer from the reception counter on the way out. It was an advertisement for a martial arts class, including an image of two black men jump kicking in what looked like white karate uniforms. As I read into it a bit more, it turns out it wasn't karate, it was actually a form of kung fu called wu shu kwan.

Hmmm.

What are the chances that a kung fu class is offered right in the hood just a few blocks from the crib? This is dope, I thought. I had my leg back in action and I took it as a sign. As they say, when the student is ready, the master will appear. I'd just walked into a new path—the path of martial arts.

THE KING OF THE PEDESTRIAN RACE

Frank Hart was a famous Haitian athlete who dominated in some of New York City's earliest foot races back in the late 1800s. Frank had mad heart; he was Black and proud of it and gave no fux. At a press conference for a race he was preparing for at Madison Square Garden, he talked his shit in spite of how hard it was for Black folks back in those days. The newspaper quoted him as saying, "I'll break those white fellows' hearts! I will—you hear me!" Frank Hart was a champion "walker" who reigned in his era, competing in six-day-long endurance challenges. These competitions were called "pedestrian races" and these walking athletes were the biggest sport icons at the time, long before modern running culture would explode almost a hundred years later in the 1980s. These pedestrian events are the unsung forerunners of the ultramarathons of today. Participants were free to run, walk, crawl, or even drag their way around a track for as many times as possible over the course of the six days. When race day came around, just as he predicted he would, Frank Hart not only won, but he set a new world record on their ass. Bro ended up walking like ninety-four miles per day for a total of 565 miles. He walked away with like twenty g's, including three stacks that he won by betting on himself! That's almost a half-million dollars in today's money. Health is wealth!

Strength Comes from Within

Our wu shu kwan class was led by two working-class Caribbean black-belt instructors, both in their midfifties—Sensei Lionel and Sensei Edward. I began training in sweatpants and T-shirts, but after a few weeks, Sensei Edward blessed me with my uniform, or *gi*— the white jacket and pants that are officially required and worn in class—and accompanied by the white belt—the beginner's rank in wu shu kwan kung fu (and many other martial-arts systems). I was in my early twenties with unstoppable energy from my new dietary discipline, and unlike back in the day when I tried to take Okinawa karate in the South City projects in Tallahassee but quit after only a few classes because I wasn't ready for the intensity, this time I was ready to put in the work.

There's usually a distinct difference in how karate and kung fu styles are taught. In a broad sense, karate has harder, straightforward movements and kung fu is usually more circular and fluid, but wu shu kwan kung fu is more similar to karate or tae kwon do than the traditional kung fu you might expect. Even the fact that we called our instructors sensei was unusual for a kung fu class, because the term sensei is a Japanese word that means teacher, whereas *sifu* is the instructor title most often used in Chinese kung fu traditions.

But nevertheless, this eclectic scenario—a Chinese martial art taught by two Caribbean senseis in a heavily Rasta neighborhood—was just the right combo I needed at the moment. It was perfect. My enthusiasm rubbed off on Afya too and she joined the dojo after a few weeks.

We did all sorts of drills, lots of leg-building stuff—a gang of kicking and horse stances until our legs wobbled from the pain, lots of push-ups, sit-ups, and stretching, fundamental striking and blocking techniques, and we also worked on kata forms—prearranged movements that drill in technical principles and teach balance in movement. We sparred a lot with our classmates, too. In one of our classes, we were instructed to get in a push-up position on our knuckles—on the hardwood floor. We had to align our wrists so we were balanced on the first two knuckles of the fist. That shit hurt. The weight of your body mashes your knuckles down into the wood and it's like a sharp, piercing kind of pain. As I think about it, it kinda reminds me of the sharp stinging pain I felt in my ankle when I had gout.

But strangely, this pain, I kind of started to enjoy it—or maybe it wasn't the pain I enjoyed, but the challenge of enduring it. Though it hurt, it also felt good to be toughening my mind and body on purpose in that way. If you've ever been under the tattoo needle, you know how it hurts but there's still a respect for the ritual of it that puts you in a state of mind to accept it. We handle pain differently when we find purpose in it. Sensei said the knuckle push-ups would help condition our fists and wrists for striking hard objects—like the skull of an attacker should we have to defend ourselves. Holding the push-up position on the knuckles also helps to strengthen the wrist so it doesn't cave in when you punch. If you've ever been in a fight and punched someone only to hurt your own wrist in the process, you know that's no fun. Unless you hold your fist and wrist in proper alignment when you strike, your own force can end up working against you. The knuckle push-ups drill strengthens that potential weakness. After some practice, and using lots of traditional Chinese herbal ointment called *dit da jow* to speed up the healing of the bruises, my knuckles eventually became desensitized to it. And my punches got stronger.

When struggling with executing my side kick right and getting frustrated about it, I told Sensei I wanted to learn how to kick better, and he gave me a jewel that I've been applying in my life in all sorts of ways ever since:

"Wanting to kick better," he said, "is not a goal; that's just a wishful statement. It's too vague." He explained that when you want to accomplish a goal, you need to be specific. A goal is stated in a way that you can measure its progress. You can't measure *better*. You have to qualify it in a way that you can actually measure. "What you *can* measure," he said, "is the strength, the speed, the height, the flexibility, or the accuracy of your kick."

Sensei continued, "To set an attainable goal, be specific. Otherwise, you are just going through the motions with no destination to reach." Decide **specifically** what you want to make progress in. How would you know if you got better unless you have a specific benchmark to measure by? Being specific allows you to focus in on your desired target.

He taught me to break down my training goals into specific areas of focus for improvement—that way I could measure progress in small increments every day. Little by little, step by step, no matter how small the progress, recognizing any improvement is motivating. Those small victories add up to winning the bigger battles. It's kind of like what I later learned are called SMART goals.

Work Smarter, Not Harder

SMART goals are an acronym; spelled out it means Specific, Measurable, Achievable, Relevant, and Timed. When we clarify and qualify our goals in these areas, they become smart goals. To this day I still set my goals in health and fitness, career, and otherwise with this in mind. At the dojo, I was getting in shape and learning a lot. Kung fu was helping me mature a lot as a person, too.

Meanwhile, by this point my hip-hop career was starting to take off. My group dead prez was signed to Loud Records and we were buzzing around the industry and in the streets of NY. At the same time, with that rise came all the trappings and temptations that come with newfound celebrity and having a li'l more paper in your pocket. It was easier than ever to relapse back to my old ways, get drunk and high all the time, find an excuse to eat bullshit on the road, and be undisciplined in all sorts of ways. On the other hand, I was trying to stand solid in my commitment to martial arts. My leg was healed and I was using it more than ever, doing hundreds if not what seemed like thousands of kicks and intense leg exercises every week. My training schedule meant adjusting to a new lifestyle of prioritizing practice time and getting more rest to have energy for my classes. That old lifestyle of late-night partying, turning up, and kicking it all the time was not gonna work if I wanted to be a serious martial-arts student. I wanted to be able to make progress in my art and handle the physical and mental demands of regular training and so I had to make choices that reflected that. I felt pulled in opposite directions at times—rapper lifestyle or martial-artist lifestyle? Slide back into distractions or stay disciplined?

People may see me as a rapper who is into these different things like martial arts and health and fitness, but it was during my wu shu kwan days that I made a fundamental shift in how I see myself. I decided that my health and fitness lifestyle would come first and the rap life second, instead of the other way around. I did my best to adjust and be a sincere student of martial arts and prioritize wellness. I wasn't perfect by any means, but making that distinction helped me put my priorities in the right order and not get sidetracked by the game...too much.

Breaking the Board

After some months, the time came around for my first rank test to earn my second rank in wu shu kwan. Though I had memorized the forms and I felt like I was ready, I was nervous, as were the rest of my classmates.

On test day, we went through our regular grueling calisthenics drills to warm up things but with even more intensity and more reps. We performed controlled sparring to show application of the techniques we'd been drilling for the last few months. We demonstrated the two katas we had learned up to that point. I was tired, but my adrenaline was carrying me through, and all was going well, I thought.

Then our senseis surprised us.

Sensei Lionel and Sensei Edward unzipped some duffel bags and pulled out short wooden planks about one and a half inches thick. They instructed us to line up in our usual ranking order. While kneeling on one knee and holding the board with two hands like an open book out in front of his chest, Sensei Edward told us that we'd each need to break through the board using the strike of our choice to complete our rank test.

What the hell? We hadn't practiced this at all. I felt caught off guard. I hadn't anticipated having to break no boards, I'm just a white belt, I thought.

Nevertheless, in the dojo when it's your turn to rock, you give it what you got.

My strike of choice was a straight punch.

When it was my turn, I focused my breathing as I'd been taught—in and out through the nose—and threw my punch with a loud yell.

"Kiyaaaa!"

Thud. Ow!

That damn board was still solid as it was before my punch.

You get two tries, or you fail.

I went to the back of the line and tried to imagine what in the hell I could do to improve by my next turn.

When I got back to the front of the line, sensei instructed me to use the kick of my choice instead of a strike.

Oh, hell naw, I thought. I *know* I can't break no board with my foot; I couldn't break it with my fist strike and I'm fresh off healing from gout. I thought, *C'mon Sensei, ain't no way*—I wouldn't dare say that out loud—*anything but kicking a board barefoot. Fuck!*

But...no time for all that drama in my head; it was my turn and so I decided to get the inevitable over with.

I decided to use the side kick. I inhaled and chambered my right knee up toward my chest, rolled my right hip over as I pivoted and balanced on the ball of my left foot and exhaled as I launched my foot at the board with everything I had!

Crack!!!

Oh shit!

The board snapped into two pieces and fell out of Sensei's grip.

I couldn't believe it! With the same foot I had gout in, that I could barely even walk on just a few months back, I had just side kicked—barefoot by the way—through a wooden board! Earning my second rank that day meant the world to me. Breaking through that board was a breakthrough on so many levels.

Get Out of Your Own Way

Have you ever had the realization that you hold yourself back from accomplishing something out of fear that you might either get hurt, embarrassed, or worse—you might reveal that you're not whatever "enough" is? That's what I was doing, I was in my own way. Breaking that board didn't change the world or anything but it did help me to change how I see myself in it. When that plank snapped, I realized at that moment that a lot of times we doubt ourselves instead of exercising our greatness because we be afraid. But we're only afraid because we don't realize how strong and capable we actually are.

You don't know your strength until it's tested.

Whether it's breaking a board, breaking free of self-sabotaging self-doubt, or breaking generational cycles, we are capable of so much more than we think. We only fail when we quit on ourselves, when we give up instead of giving it all we got. Life is the greatest sensei, and there are many things it will put in front of us to test us and teach us. We have to get out of our own way and trust the universe and keep kicking until we break through whatever the test may be.

Over the years, martial arts has helped me realize there's so much more to physical training than meets the eye. There's a lot of *meaning* in movement. I started to look at fitness in a deeper way, and to move with more confidence and trust in the process because of all the diamonds I found in the discipline of the physical challenges. I learned to not be afraid to fail at first, or a number of times, because those attempts have valuable game in them that is needed to succeed. I realized that not only was I learning self-defense and getting in great shape from the physical movements, but I was also learning deep insights about what I'm made of and how a lot of the times I be in my own way. Through training, we reveal more of ourselves to ourselves. When I first signed up to take kung fu, I was just excited to be able to be physically active again, but what I thought was just gonna be physical exercise, I soon realized was enhancing my life way beyond the dojo. It was strengthening my character. When you become aware that your exercise is a vehicle for self-understanding and it reveals keys on how to live your life better, fitness takes on a whole new level of meaning and significance. You start to realize you need it, it's not optional. It has to be a part of your life.

African Martial Arts

African drums always energized the room and set the tone for my *ile ijala* classes—a rare African martial art system that Afya, several of our friends, and I started taking after a couple years of training in wu shu kwan kung fu. Our instructor, Master Woza Vega, trained us all at the Marcus Garvey Community Center just five blocks north on Nostrand Avenue from the World Fitness Center. Woza was a raw foodist with the build of a professional running back and wore neat dreadlocks and a five o'clock shadow–styled beard. My very first encounter with him was actually before we started training full time at the Marcus Garvey Center, at a boxing gym in Downtown Brooklyn on Fourth Street and Flatbush. He'd extended an invitation for us to take a free-trial class and get a sample of what his style of teaching was like.

When you entered the building, you had to climb up a steep flight of stairs to the gym's entrance, where there was a pull-up bar welled into a cubby space facing the door. Afya and I put our stuff down and expected to take off our shoes and get started. But before starting class, Woza said we had to "warm up" on the pull-up bar to *earn* our entrance.

Guess how many pull-ups he told us we had to do?

For real, take a guess.

How many do you think? Ten? Twenty? Twenty-five?

Can you believe this dude said we had to complete two hundred pull-ups in order to start class? And yes, Afya, too! Mind you, this was just to start class! This was the warm-up! I was intimidated; I hadn't done two hundred pull-ups in my whole life if you added 'em all up together, let alone in one session. Honestly, I probably hadn't even done twenty pull-ups in total since the mandatory PE evaluations back in elementary school. Now here I was looking at what seemed like a mountain of two hundred pull-ups in front of me.

But I had to remind myself that mindset matters. That's when the lessons in fortitude I'd been learning in kung fu kicked in again and reinspired me. I knew the only strategy to get the shits done was with lots of breaks over multiple sets, so I just said fuck it and got to it, alternating sets with Afya. I surprised myself by banging out like eighteen in my first clip. Not bad. I took a breather to shake my arms out and after Afya muscled out her first set, we both looked at each other like, "Whose idea was this?" and laughed out loud.

Then we took turns banging out another set. We'd rest a minute or so and stretch out our arms and then hit the bar again, hanging and pulling, hanging and pulling 'til failure. Over and over, sometimes doing only four or five per set, but we kept at it. Every time I thought, *I don't have no more in me to keep going*, I'd think about how disappointing giving up would feel and I'd jump back on that bar with more resolve to get 'em done. After short breaks, somehow again and again we were able to jump back on the bar and pump out more. Over and over—little by little—until finally, miraculously, two hundred raggedy fucking pull-ups—done!

Sweating like rain, we clapped it up for ourselves and claimed our victory. "We finished!" we told Woza, feeling accomplished, excited, and exhausted, and expecting to be celebrated for our efforts. He simply nodded and said, "Good you're warmed up, grab the jump ropes."

And like that, we got started.

I was really impressed by the level of physical skill and power Woza demonstrated. He would toss students around effortlessly, showing us the effectiveness of different techniques. At one point, he took on three students in the boxing ring at once and had them tripping over their own feet and knocking into each other like the three stooges. His form, footwork, speed, precision, flow, and Afrocentric perspective really inspired us to want to learn from him.

With my homey's help in pulling it all together, I connected the dots for Woza to train us at the Marcus Garvey Center. I knew the Cameroonian brother Ametu—who owned the space and was a true-blue Garveyite—would surely be open to hosting an African-centered self-defense class in the community. It was a gritty space (to put it nicely) that needed a lot of work, but Ametu was a community visionary and this diamond in the rough represented his hopes for our community, and there was no way he was going to turn away our crew of young folks who were trying to bring something positive to our hood.

Sprouts and Water

When we began our training at the center, Woza taught us that *ile ijala* means "house of the warrior" and is both a physical and spiritual-based system of West African origin mixed with his own athletic expertise and sauce. Each class began with a libation, where we poured water to honor the ancestors and align our hearts and minds with the sacredness of our training. Then, three times a week from 6:00 to 9:00 p.m., we banged out. With the drum rhythms pulsating in the background, we trained and we sweat. We didn't have uniforms or belts like traditional Asian martial arts do in ijala. I usually just wore an old T-shirt, my old wu shu kwan gi pants, or some sweats and my Asics wrestling shoes—we never trained barefoot.

We worked on a wide range of techniques and drills—punches, kicks, footwork, elbow and knee strikes, Western boxing–style strikes, slipping, bobbing, weaving, and parrying, and lots of stretching and full-contact sparring.

Woza also gave us plenty of long but insightful lectures. There were times where me and other students would lock eyes, wondering how long before we'd get to the action, but there would be other times where we'd be doing so much, we would be wishing for a lecture so we could take a break. Woza also gave us culturally relevant reading assignments—we had to study *Stolen Legacy* by George G. M. James and memorize the ten cardinal virtues that were the foundation of ancient Egypt's mystery schools. *Stolen Legacy* talked about how much of the philosophies that enlightened Europe came from African culture. Egypt was the Harvard of the world in ancient times, and it was in their mystery schools that they taught groundbreaking insights into the principles of life and nature through spiritual rituals, initiations, and rites of passage. Our three- and often four-hour-long classes were enlightening and grueling and so much fun. Some days we'd do one thousand kicks or five hundred punches or both just to begin class. It was beast mode. Woza also required us to study first aid. We were quizzed on making tourniquets and other survival skills. If we weren't on point, we'd pay for it in perspiration.

Woza was all about teaching us the "sprouts and water," his remix of the phrase "bread and butter"—meaning the basic fundamentals of fitness, not just martial-arts techniques. We did insane amounts of calisthenics for strength work and endurance and he really stressed flexibility, too. We devoted almost thirty minutes or more per class to flexibility drills. There was one stretching exercise where you'd be on your back with your butt and legs up against the wall stretched open into a wide V. The aim was to just hang there, breathe and let gravity pull down on your legs and open your hips into a side split, or as close as you could manage.

The old rugs on the floor stank; they were mildewed and disgusting and you never wanted to let your skin touch them. You'd be laying there looking up at the ceiling while in the deep stretch and the smell from those rugs would be horrible. But we just accepted it as a part of the training. I remember my hamstrings always felt tight at first, but after ten minutes or so, they'd start to loosen up causing my legs to sink downward little by little, relaxing and opening up more and more. Woza would come around and push down on your legs even more to maximize the stretch. I hated and loved it. But it stamped in my mind that flexibility is something you have to take the time to develop and maintain.

Woza and I spent a lot of time together outside of class training and building as well. We'd finish class, then walk the few blocks back to my basement apartment on Dean Street and we'd continue to train and build some more. Because of my fondness for Bruce Lee and my dedication as a student at that time, Woza nicknamed me "Black Bruce" and often whenever I'd be sparring, he'd call me that for motivation. Afya would tease me, saying I was the teacher's pet. But in truth, I was never a natural talent in martial arts by any means. I still struggled with getting my mind and body to coordinate together and even though I had learned a lot of the basics in wu shu kwan, and I practiced all the time, I was still not as competent in my body as I wanted to be in my head. But still, I loved how the training made me feel. Afya's form, on the other hand, was amazing; her kicks were the best in our class. She was a natural, but her consistency helped her develop even quicker. At home, she would always be stretching. She's always been rubbing off on me in positive ways.

As beast mode as our regular weekly classes were, our advancement tests were even more epic. Our testing process was like a rite of passage in itself. That's actually what Woza called them. The rites test took place over a whole week on multiple days, and these were four-hour-plus classes. Ijala had me in great shape and it was inspiring my life in so many ways.

You may not have the time to devote to three- and four-hour-long classes like we did at the time, but you know what? We find the time for what we are passionate about. People spend a lot of time in front of the TV every evening or scrolling for hours on phones, so it's really about prioritizing the time we have to get the most out of it.

While all this was happening, I of course was still pursuing my career as a hip-hop artist. After I produced our debut single "Hip Hop," I was working on writing out my ideas for the video treatment for the song, and we selected director Brian Beletic to help execute the vision. He loved it when I told him my idea to include our ile ijala class in the mix. The group martial-arts performance you see in that video was shot at the Marcus Garvey Center where we actually trained, and those are some of my classmates demonstrating real drills that we would do in class.

Cultural Movement

The more we understand, the deeper and more meaningful will be our contact with all that is around us.

—*Bruce Lee*

Years later when I moved to Atlanta, I explored *kupigana ngumi*—the umbrella Kiswahili term for African martial arts as a whole—and I got to study another African martial-arts system: egbe ogun, taught by Master Balogun, whom I also helped publish a now-out-of-print text on egbe ogun called *African Martial Arts*.

Training in egbe ogun was a deep dive into the unsung African roots of martial arts and African spirituality. We trained to recordings of African drumming just as we did in ijala, which is pretty much standard in African fighting arts, but egbe ogun differed from ijala in that there was more emphasis on ground fighting, grappling, and wrestling techniques. Balogun didn't want us to be rigid and stiff and machine-like; he encouraged us to appreciate and use our African originality and flavor to our advantage. We were encouraged to tap into our "soul," our own natural flair and sauce when sparring and executing our techniques. "Africans don't just play basketball or make music or anything in the standard old tight-ass way," he explained. "Everything we do we add our own swag to it and martial arts is no exception." He encouraged us to use all the instinctive broken rhythm and organic sense of athletic timing that comes so naturally in African expression.

You could call what he was referring to our *rhythmic* intelligence. You know that style and finesse you see the youngbloods in the hood demonstrate on the basketball courts who are super nice with their footwork, and their feints and fakes and tricks. *That.* It was about keeping those cultural mannerisms alive in our practice. He said that was an advantage against any opponent that is rhythmically challenged.

We also learned about martial connections to *orishas*, which are considered divine expressions of natural powers in the Yoruba tradition, and in particular, we learned about the orisha known as Ogun—the principle that represents war, creativity and destruction, clearing the way, and iron. Not just the iron that makes weapons, or railroad spikes and things like that, but also the iron in our own blood and how it all connects on a supernatural, ancestral level. Egbe ogun was more than fitness, more than self-defense; it brought spiritual ritual to the physical training. Our breath connects us with nature and the DNA of our ancestors and their wisdom and strength is literally in our blood. I came to understand that those connections can be accessed through our physical training practice.

Not only were we pouring water in libation to begin our classes, I realized that the sweat pouring out of our pores is also a powerful form of libation.

Culture can be a powerful vehicle in finding your fitness. It doesn't have to be your native culture per se but taking an interest in the cultural roots of whatever physical training practice you have will definitely make it more meaningful.

Enter The Dragon: Jeet Kune Do

Sifu Ralph Mitchell's Universal Defense Systems (UDS) is a school of martial arts that offers an eclectic mix of fighting styles and has been home to several state champions in mixed martial arts, stick fighting, praying mantis kung fu, and more. After searching far and wide, it was the best—and actually only—reputable place I could find back then in the early 2000s in NYC that offered classes in jeet kune do concepts—the martial arts system that Bruce Lee personally developed and taught.

As a martial artist and as a role model, Bruce Lee has probably had the biggest influence on my evolution as a man that any one person has had on my life outside of my immediate family or maybe Malcolm X. I had seen all the movies and watched a ton of documentaries and read many books about Bruce Lee, including a compilation of his own writings on his personal philosophy of martial arts called the *Tao of Jeet Kune Do*. So, when I applied to UDS and was accepted as a student, *you already know I leaped at the opportunity.*

It was an epic commute to and from the Universal Defense Systems school three to four times a week. UDS was located in Canarsie, a kind of far out area of Brooklyn, and to get there from my crib in Crown Heights, I had to take the subway and transfer at two different junctures, then take a bus. Then, when I got off at my bus stop, I had to walk another mile to get to the school. But it meant so much to me to study Bruce's art firsthand, so I happily did what I had to do.

The thing that stood out right away about the way the whole UDS school operated was the nontraditional approach. Jeet kune do or JKD wasn't structured like conventional martial arts are structured. Traditionally, martial arts, especially Asian martial arts, are taught the same way they have been taught for thousands of years—to preserve the tradition and the way the original founders of the style first instructed. But jeet kune do, which means "the way of the intercepting fist," is more of an open, living system of combat concepts. There was no rigid traditional pageantry to follow. We didn't wear any uniforms, we didn't have belts to indicate rank, and we wore sweats and street shoes in class.

Sifu Mitchell is a legend himself and it was truly an honor to study with him for the two years I got to train there. He was a combat veteran who served in Vietnam, a master of many martial arts, and had a decorated career as a tournament champion in both forms and fighting. Sifu was an expert in southern praying mantis kung fu; he trained in boxing under Victor Valle Sr. and Fred Corritone. He trained under gurus Paul Vunak and Thomas Cruse, and became a senior full instructor in their Progressive Fighting Systems. He held black belts in judo and the doce pares system of eskrima—a stick-fighting art from the Philippines, similar to kali. He had been training partners with other legends in the martial-arts world such as Soke Li'l John Davis, Shidoshi Ron Van Clief, and learned JKD concepts directly from Dan Inosanto, one of Bruce Lee's top students.

Sifu Mitchell encouraged us in the same spirit that Bruce Lee had taught his students, to explore and use what works best for the natural attributes of our bodies, temperaments, and abilities. The way we were sampling from all sorts of combat arts and influences reminded me of hip-hop in how we sample different musical influences to make our own unique music. There's an organic kinship in the mentality of hip-hop and what Bruce innovated with JKD. I felt right at home.

Sifu encouraged us to study Miyamoto Musashi's classic *The Book of Five Rings*, which details the legendary Japanese swordsman's strategies and insights on combat. He particularly emphasized that we sit with the chapters on one-on-one combat. We studied eskrima/kali stick fighting and learned the doce pares twelve-strikes system with the double sticks. We worked on the forms using a single stick, double sticks, machetes, umbrellas, even rolled-up magazines. We learned footwork techniques from a French martial art called savate and incorporated fencing strategies in our toolbox of kicking techniques. We drilled Western-boxing basics—straight lead, jab, left cross, upper cuts—but unlike the usual left lead in boxing, JKD uses a southpaw, right-hand lead, so we would work on alternating the lead to be prepared for any position in which you might find yourself in a real fight.

We worked on wing chun concepts like centerline theory, sticky hands, and more. Sifu showed us a range of elbow, shoulder, and wrist strikes, eye gouges from praying mantis, and we even worked on headbutts. Anything and everything goes. We worked on our ground game too, drilling basic jujitsu submissions, controls, and escapes. Even when I'd come home with huge blood bubbles and blisters on my arms from stick training, or with my ego bruised after getting dusted by one of my amazing sparring partners, again and again I wore those blisters and ass whippings like badges of honor. That three-train ride to bus ride to one-mile walk commute there and back three times a week was some of the best time spent in my life.

Sometimes you've got to go outside of your comfort zone (or zip code) to find your fitness.

Jeet kune do was a crash course in simplicity, directness, and freedom. Every session was unique in some way, always emphasizing key principles as the guide and encouraging personal freedom as the expression. No limitation. Our range of tools and techniques came from all kinds of sources. Bruce Lee's mantra of taking what's useful, discarding what's not, and adding what's essentially your own sums up the JKD approach so well. That "principled yet free" approach has stuck with me over the years and it continues to influence how I approach my personal fitness training and my life in general.

Military Minded

As a young kid, long before the streets became my battlefield, and before I became politicized by the Black Power movement, I was fascinated with the military and I fantasized that I'd grow up and join; believe it or not, I was dead set on becoming an Army Ranger. Those who knew me at that time would tell you I was obsessed with soldier life, reading everything I could get my hands on about military history, culture, and tactics.

My pops was a sergeant in the Air Force who served in Vietnam as an electronic tech, repairing communication systems in war-damaged aircraft. I grew up looking at black-and-white pictures in our family photo albums from when he was stationed in Thailand. The uniforms, the camaraderie, the world adventure, his Thai girlfriend, it all inspired me. I thought it was inevitable that I'd grow up and be a soldier, too. I hiked and foraged and sketched out my own maps of the seven acres of surrounding woodlands we lived on that my pops purchased for only $5,000 when I was a toddler. My friends and I had BB-gun wars and firework battles and used socks for boxing gloves for hand-to-hand combat training, acting out our strategies and fantasies to become soldiers. I was super ready to enlist; I even sent out handwritten letters to the Army in middle school to ask if I could drop out of school and join early.

It wasn't until much later, in high school, that I read Malcolm X's powerful autobiography and later learned about Muhammad Ali's defiant and honorable stance against being drafted for the Vietnam War that I woke up out of the path I was headed. Malcolm X's and Muhammad Ali's bravery, honesty, and political awareness helped me realize how I was to the political aspects of what it means to be a soldier in the American military-industrial complex. Just because I respected the soldiers' disciplined lifestyle didn't mean I had to cosign the politics behind the war machine.

I'm glad they woke me up, and I ultimately decided to go in a different direction, but nevertheless, Bruce Lee's ever-relevant mantra of "taking what's useful and discarding what's not," still applies. I've learned you can be military minded in getting things done effectively in your personal life without necessarily signing up for military service. And I also respect the fact that there are many people who have chosen to join for their own reasons, and it's been a huge benefit to their lives. I salute those who've been able to be of better service to their families and communities because of their military training and education. Geronimo Pratt, who taught the Black Panther Party defensive maneuvers that he learned on combat tours in Vietnam, is a wonderful example. Those early years of being an army enthusiast planted a lot of seeds for me that have stuck with me to this day in how I think and live.

The wisdom that Sensei taught me in wu shu kwan about having SMART goals is an example of something that is also a hallmark of the military tradition: *setting and maintaining measurable fitness standards.*

Standards of Fitness

In military speak, "SOP" stands for standard operating procedures. SOPs are guidelines that lay out what is required for carrying out a particular mission or task, how to go about it, and how success will be measured. It's a systematized way to provide soldiers with a set of standardized instructions that get desired results. We can all use standards to live by that will hold us accountable to our goals. When it comes to finding your fitness and building out your own training regimen, the military has a powerhouse of exercise information to take advantage of.

The Army physical fitness assessment test, or APFT, is a great example. It was first developed in 1858 at the United States Military Academy. The test is designed to ensure the maintenance of a base level of physical fitness that is considered essential for every soldier. The current standard that was instituted in 1980 is a three-part test of calisthenics—push-ups, sit-ups, and a two-mile run testing arm strength, core strength, and cardiovascular endurance, performed in that order. Soldiers are allowed a minimum of ten minutes and a maximum of twenty minutes of rest between events, so long as all three events are completed within two hours. The maximum score a Soldier can achieve on the test is three hundred points. Soldiers must earn a minimum score of at least sixty points on each event and an overall score of at least 180 points to qualify for the standard.

You can try it out and see where you measure up:

- You have two minutes to do as many push-ups as you can.
- Then, you have two minutes to do as many sit-ups as you can.
- And finally, you have to complete a two-mile run.

It's a performance test that indicates a soldier's ability to physically perform and handle their own body weight.

We don't all have to join the military to get in shape, but we don't have to completely reinvent the wheel either. Just as the military uses fitness standards, so can civilians.

One of my homies, Pree, is an Air Force vet. He's always in great shape; living in Arizona, he does monthly timed runs in the desert to maintain his own personal cardio standards.

On social media, I've become a huge fan of an elder Rasta sister who lives in Hawaii. She always posts footage from her daily ten-mile morning walks in the lush green island surroundings, while bumping my *Workout II* album. Her positive spirit and the joy of movement she displays in her posts always brighten my day.

I created a super simple five-minute workout for both my mom and mother-in-law for their morning routines, where they do five consecutive one-minute exercises like squats, light dumbbells, arm raises, crunches, and a minute of deep breathing. It's short, sweet, and effective. The aim is to go sixty seconds nonstop from exercise to exercise and in just five minutes, they're done. They each get a nice full body charge, and both have expressed that they enjoy and look forward to it because it gives them more energy and helps them feel good at the beginning of the day.

Finding Your Fitness

Those are just a few of the infinite ways there are to keep an active fitness standard in our lives. It's never one-size-fits-all. It's about your personal standard of fitness, your interests, needs, and goals, and set-ting standards that help keep you doing the activities that allow you to feel how you want to feel in your life. If we want to feel good and be strong then that's the standard we set for ourselves to encourage us to stick to the discipline. Sure, we might all slack off from time to time, but we don't want to get so slack our lives become full of excuses instead of fulfillment. Nobody don't really want to feel chronically tired, out of shape, and weak. That's not a standard to aspire to; that's settling for way less than what life can be. We want to feel energized, strong, and powerful. We want to have standards that allow us to live life to the fullest. We want to strive for having fitness in our lives, families, and communities as the standard, not the exception.

To that end, I believe we should take the "fit" in fitness liter-ally. As in, it needs to be *custom fit* to your particular needs, your preferences, what's practical, and what sits right with your cultural values. There's the fit in the sense of physical fitness standards like in the military and then there is the definition of "fit" as in what "fits right for you"—what suits and complements you best. When some-thing "fits," it's designed with the user in mind and caters to their specifics. If an outfit "fits" it means it accommodates and accents your frame and "suits you well." Your fitness should fit just as well. And you've got to be willing to try different things on, because sometimes it takes some trial and error to find your fit.

Hoop Dreams

Back in high school, I don't even know how I managed to make the team. I'd only tried out because every time I happened to be in the gym, the coach would keep asking me, "*Why don't you try out for the bas-ketball team?*" I mean, I was tall, Black, and skinny, so I guess I fit the stereotype, but I ain't really know shit about no basketball. I played for fun every so often with my cousins on the courts in the hood and talked my little shit, but I wasn't no be-on-no-real-basketball-team material by no means. I didn't even like watching it on TV. But coach kept badgering me about tryouts and when he mentioned we'd get to travel for out-of-town games I got really interested. I decided to go for it, and what do you know, I fucked around and made the damn team. I was hype at first but then my uniform fit me funny 'cause I was so tall and so skinny. That shit was too big and too small at the same damn time. I just knew I looked goofy as hell.

Our first game of the season was an away game. I had been keeping the bench warm for the whole game so far, and we were already in the second half. I was sitting there daydreaming—or probably rapping under my breath back then—but whatever I was doing, I wasn't paying attention to the game, that was fasho. All of a sudden, our coach called out my jersey number.

Oh shit! That's me!

My heart was beating fast as hell and I was about to get my first taste of live-game action.

Picture a tall skinny teenager in an awkward-fitting uniform with big feet. That was me on the sidelines, green as hell, and nervous but excited. I stepped on the court and my teammate checked the ball in with a pass to me. In the next few moments my career in basketball was decided.

Dribbling a couple of times, I took two steps and paused at half-court with the opposing team's guard a few feet in front of me, trying his best to anticipate my next move. I looked down court at my teammates who were all vying to get open for a pass.

I looked at the basket.

Now mind you, I had already taken all the steps I could legally take, or the ref would call traveling.

In the heat of that moment, the way I saw it, I had two options: I could just pass the ball to an open teammate and then run down the

court, run the plays we drilled at practice for a few uneventful minutes until the coach yanked me back out of the game, and I'd go back
to warming the bench for the rest of the night...

Or—

I looked back at the basket.

Everything around me went silent and I had a wild, impulsive
thought: What if I were to actually shoot and make this shot from
here? Man, I'd be legendary. The crowd would go wild. The chicks
would be like, *Who is that?* My teammates would be high-fiving me
like I was fucking Jordan. I'd be on my way to the NBA!

"This is my chance," I told myself, delusional.

So, what did I do? I shot that shit...

Air ball.

Turnover.

The player from the other team quickly scored an easy layup off
that goofy shit I'd just pulled, and I hadn't even realized I was still
standing in the same spot like a mannequin watching it all go down
until coach snapped me out of my foolishness yelling, **"What the fuck
are you doing? Get out of there!"**

And that, my friend, was the beginning and end of my basketball career.
Basketball, goofy uniform and all, was definitely not a good fit for me.

All jokes aside, that experience left me feeling like I just wasn't
cut out for sports in general and it took me a while to recover from,
unlearn, and let go of that limiting belief I took on about myself.

And my first foray into karate, years before, hadn't gone much better
either. As a little kid, I had emulated Bruce Lee moves in the living room
for as long as I could remember, and you couldn't tell me I wasn't no
little nappy-headed ninja. But my first actual attempt at formally learning martial arts was *Okinawa* karate when I was about ten years old.

Sensei Edward X was a street-smart Black Muslim with a gold-
tooth smile who held classes on the south side of Tallahassee in the
South City projects. To say the training was tough and demanding

is an understatement. I don't know what the hell I thought I'd been doing back at home, but this shit was crazy. I'd never done so many kicks and punches over and over in a row like he was commanding us to do. My white belt kept coming loose and falling down. My nose was running, and it was hard to breathe. The intensity of all the physical drills would make my stomach queasy, my head dizzy and hot, and I felt disoriented like I was going to throw up and pass out. The reality of all that hard work burst my little karate fantasy bubble quicker than a motherfucker. After just one summer, I decided flat out, I ain't cut out for no karate, and I quit.

It's so important when we're striving to find our fitness that we don't let the activities that don't seem like a good fit stop us from continuing to believe in our ability to find something that does.

It took me years to finally find my flow in fitness. It wasn't until I was almost twenty-two years old or so before I found my groove in martial arts. There's no one way that works for everybody and sometimes you've got to try out a bunch of stuff before you find your fitness, but the great thing is there's mad options to explore. A lifter might not want to run a marathon. A yogi might not wanna lift heavy weights. And at the same time, a runner or a bodybuilder might want to also explore the added benefit of cross-training with yoga or meditation. You might like training solo; somebody else might thrive in classes or team sports or water sports. There are infinite ways you can go about living a fitness lifestyle.

My encouragement to you is to explore, play the field so to speak, and establish your own fitness standards based on what fits your preferences and what's accessible for you. If you were the character Akeem from the movie *Coming to America*, I'd tell you to go and sow your royal oats before you marry the wrong girl. Seriously though, a lasting fitness practice is tailor fit to *benefit* you, and it can change. It don't have to be one thing; it can be many different ways you can bang out. It don't matter what somebody else's fitness looks like, finding *your* fitness means discovering a custom fit practice that you rock with. It matters, because if the exercise practice you choose ain't a good fit, you are going to quit. Simple as that. At the end of the day, the best exercise program for you is the one you'll actually do. That's when you know you've found your right fit.

When your fitness practice fits in well with your life and who you are, it's more likely to stick.

The Four Pillars

There are some core principles that should always be part of a well-rounded fitness practice. I call them the four pillars: strength, flexibility, endurance, and vitality. You might remember those same four pillars from when we were discussing mental and emotional fitness in earlier chapters. Fitness is fitness, mind and body—it's all connected. As long as your physical training incorporates a range of activities that exercise those same four pillars in your rotation, you'll have a solid regimen.

You may find a sport or activity that does it all for you. Dancing, swimming, and surfing come to mind as possible one-stop-shops that incorporate all four pillars, but there's no limit to all the training modalities and fitness activities you can explore to exercise one or more of the pillars.

You can hit the weights or do calisthenics for strength training.

Yoga, Pilates, and stretching are great practices for flexibility.

Distance running, jumping rope, and sparring are a few of many ways to work on endurance.

Qigong, yoga, and pranayama are good examples of vitality exercises that emphasize internal energy development and deep mindful breathing to support the longevity of your inner body and organ systems.

Today, I still strive to do a range of exercises in my personal workout routines that touch on strength, flexibility, endurance, and vitality year-round. This way, I'm free to customize my workout and mix things up and avoid too much monotony. I know by incorporating some strength training, both lifting weights and body-weight exercises, some endurance work, some stretching for flexibility, and some qigong and breath work mixed in there, my fitness practice is covering all the fundamental bases.

The intense focus of the martial-arts lifestyle fit my personality well and I think that's why it was so fulfilling for me over the decade of practice I put in. It provided practical training for self-defense, which I value. The calisthenics, stretching, and sparring improved my strength, flexibility, and endurance and the cultural and philosophical insights fed my vital need to keep learning and growing as a person. Martial arts and working out in general have meant so much in my life.

Finding Meaning through Movement

In psychology, *meaning making* is the process of how we make sense of our lives. It's the *why* behind what we do. With any moves we make in life, if they really mean something to us, we move differently, we move with purpose. It's no different with literal exercise movements— you're not just moving your body; you are finding meaning in the movement and experiencing *why your physical practice matters in your life*.

Meaning is about how things correspond to others and fit within a coherent framework, their impact, role, and significance within the whole. When your fitness becomes a commitment in your life, you aren't just going through the motions anymore, you're not just forcing yourself to exercise, you are doing it because of what it means to you. **You are moving with meaning.**

Say for example, you're tasked with carrying some heavy-ass weights up twenty flights of stairs. You could do that if you absolutely had to, right? Maybe? Probably! It might not be fun, but if you had to, it could get done.

But why would you do that? What would make you want to do that?

Now say those heavy weights are instead heavy bags of groceries, and the elevator is broken in your building, and the reason you are carrying them is to help an elder up to the top floor.

Does that mean something more to you when there is purpose or service involved? Does helping the elder inspire or motivate you to want to carry that weight?

The first scenario is just work for work's sake, it's just a chore. But the grocery-bag scenario puts the work in a context that gives it a more significant purpose. Carrying groceries for Grandma has more meaning, right?

You've heard the story of the mom who lifts the car to free her child from under it. Purpose can summon strength we don't even know we have.

When we move with meaning behind it, we tap into another level of our energy and potential.

Bruce Lee was definitely about bringing that kind of "emotional content" to your training and fighting. He thought about "killer instinct" in that way. He said when you spar you better imagine that the opponent in front of you has threatened your mama or your kids' lives. He advocated bringing that real kind of emotional X factor to your practice so that your nervous system and your spirit and whole being are engaged in your practice. I think his expertise as an actor leant that insight into how he made his training so realistic. We want to bring that emotional content into our fitness activities and use it to our advantage. Let purpose turn up your intensity. The more realistic we make our training, the more we can rely on our training in real situations.

I've taken yoga classes, and a lot of them will start with deep breathing and the instructor will invite the class to take a moment to set an intention for their practice. Bringing a sense of purpose to the mat gives you an opportunity to tap into something that inspires your effort in a meaningful way, so you're not just chugging through a chore, you are carrying groceries for Grandma, you are protecting a loved one, you are sweating for a significant reason in your life. And that's always going to be more powerful than just going through the motions.

The more something matters to us, the stronger we become. Strength comes from within.

The word *calisthenics* actually comes from two ancient Greek words. *Kalos* and *sthenos*. "Kalos" means beautiful and "sthenos" means strength. Strength can be measured in muscle force, power, and movement, but beauty is measured in the mind and by what the experience means to the participant. We have both muscle and mind, so we are not made just to move, we are made to move with insight, purpose, and meaning. For me, exercise is a physical discipline, spiritual medicine, and therapeutic play all intertwined in one. Your fitness practice doesn't have to look like mine or anyone else's. You have to exercise *your* greatness. You can build your own custom-fit fitness practices according to what has meaning for you. When it feels meaningful to you, that means you've found your *why* and that's what you are going to need to stick with it. Have fun, try shit, mix it up. Exercise your greatness.

CHAPTER 10

Going the Distance

> Most people want to skip the process, not knowing
> that when you skip steps, you miss the lessons. If you
> start small and build on what you have, you can con-
> tinue to multiply that into something greater, while
> picking up all of the valuable lessons along the way.
>
> —*Nipsey Hussle*

Martial arts were my primary fitness practice for over ten years. It provided me with priceless lessons in personal growth and self-development. It made me a healthier and better person in all aspects—physically, mentally, and spiritually. But after a decade of that focus, while simultaneously juggling my dead prez career and touring nonstop, moving from Brooklyn to Atlanta, and starting my own entrepreneurial ventures, attending regular martial-arts classes became less of a priority. With all the to-dos and shifts in my life I didn't keep up with my self-defense training as much as I once had.

I still practiced my basic self-defense techniques in our basement to maintain my core skills, and to teach my son Twezo a thing or two here and there, but I was no longer taking formal classes. I was in my thirties and starting to feel kinda rusty, like an old boxer who hadn't been in the ring for a while, when it just so happened that I found this gritty, old-school boxing gym that inspired my path to go in a whole new direction.

As part of our family traditions, I've curated and coordinated our own rite-of-passage experiences to ensure my sons learn essential life skills on their way to manhood. We believe taking care of ourselves and being able to protect ourselves are fundamental rights and responsibilities of every person, and so one of those required life skills is self-defense training. Twezo had taken shotokan karate as a youth and a bit of egbe ogun with me, but boxing was the first martial art he chose for himself. He was around ten years old when he began training at Atlanta Art of Boxing.

Atlanta Art of Boxing was a gritty, nostalgic sweathouse with cracked leather heavy bags wrapped in silver duct tape swinging to and fro like big slabs of beef in a meat house. Vintage posters of the greats like Ali, Holyfield, Mayweather, and Hearns covered the dingy cinder-block walls. Old, dusty workout equipment cluttered every corner. The locker room reeked of sweat, urine, and Lysol. Speed-bag stations and pull-up bars flanked two giant boxing rings at the center of the room.

My role for my son (and "neighborhood" nephew who rolled with us) was initially just as support to drive them to and from the boxing gym, but their coach Johnny Gant—a legend in his own right who had faced off and held his own with Sugar Ray Leonard in his prime—recruited me from the sidelines and put me to work as their volunteer training assistant. I never want to be the kind of parent doing too much interfering with the coach's role, but once he gave me the green light, I enjoyed assisting. I would even join in and sweat with them as they learned to skip rope, got the hang of the speed bag and the heavy bag, worked on calisthenics, used focus mitts, and practiced footwork.

TRAINING FOR DISTANCE

Boxing has been around for centuries, with the earliest recorded evidence of boxing dating back to 3000 BC in ancient Sumer. "Roadwork" is how boxers often refer to the running that is a part of their training regimen. It's rooted in the culture of the sport. Roadwork is low-intensity, steady-state running for long durations. Muhammad Ali started each morning with prayer and outdoor roadwork. Running was a core part of his training. Along with lots of sparring, running helped Ali have the endurance to maintain stamina through fifteen rounds. Roadwork provided him a key advantage as a heavyweight.

Boxing Inspiration

Boxing gyms are full of character. There's a distinct culture of perseverance and hard work in the air. I met a lot of upcoming fighters there. One female fighter they called Goose trained there. Imagine a woman who looks like a Colombian Halle Berry but hits like fucking Mike Tyson. She was phenomenal. I met another good brother who had both his young sons training there and they were both really nice with it, great technical skills and positive, humble attitudes. Inspiring guys. There was another boxer who went by the name Bones, and one of the first things I noticed was how ripped dude's abs were. I admired his work ethic; he would be drenched in sweat all the time and seemed to really push himself at all the stations around the gym. He was hungry.

Bones was from Brooklyn and recognized me from dead prez, and so we connected on that level and we'd chop it from time to time when we each were resting in between the training buzzer rounds. We mostly reminisced about the "old Brooklyn," before gentrification, and the golden era of hip-hop. He'd always ask me my thoughts on different emcees and hip-hop culture and I'd ask him about his craft of boxing.

One day I asked him, "Bro what's your regimen like to get the level of definition you have in your abs? Your shit is crazy."

He countered my question with a question, "How much do you run?"

I hadn't even thought about running in a fitness sense for as long as I could remember. I was in my midthirties and all my fitness practice in recent years had been martial-arts classes and body-weight calisthenic workouts. And as I said, at that particular time it had been a while since I had been in a steady martial-arts class. So, other than the jump ropes and the drilling at the boxing gym, which was more father and son time than anything else, my cardio left a lot to be desired.

I said, "I don't really run at all."

Bones gave me a challenge that would have an unexpected domino effect in my life. He was like, "You have to get your cardio up to burn the layer of fat on your midsection so the muscle can show through." He said a lot of guys is too lazy to run, "but if you do like I'm telling you and start banging out your runs it will help you chisel up." He said to start small and aim for five to ten minutes of continuous running and see how that feels. Then build up to twenty to thirty minutes.

Bones said, "Before you know it, you'll be running forty-five minutes to an hour no problem."

Run for an hour, nonstop? That's some impossible-sounding shit, I thought. But something about how he broke down those incremental benchmarks made the impossible feel attainable. Smart goals. I've been here before. This was the kind of impossible that had my name on it.

That same week I started running.

Roadwork

I started out like Bones said, setting my phone alarm for five minutes. I figured I could handle that because our jump-rope routine at the gym was three, three-minute rounds and I was used to that by then. That first run went cool and wasn't so bad. The next day or so I went out again for a little longer, maybe eight minutes or so. Next time maybe ten. But after I hit that ten-minute mark, my body would feel like I was overheating or something and my mind would flood with doubt and I would stop. I felt like I had hit my limit. I was starting to think I might have bit off more than I could chew with this running shit. How on earth would it be possible for me to keep running for a whole hour, nonstop? I couldn't see it.

My martial-arts lessons kicked in once again. I remembered days I'd dug deep and squeezed out two hundred pull-ups when I couldn't have fathomed it beforehand. Or other times when I had managed to crank out a thousand kicks or hundreds of punches on a regular basis in ijala. I had proven to myself again and again that no matter how hard it seems, anything can be accomplished when you commit and put in the work, and this running shit was no different, I reassured myself. I decided that I really, really wanted to see how awesome it would feel in my body to run for a whole hour nonstop. I became positively *obsessed* with that goal.

Day in and day out, little by little over those next few weeks I stayed at it. Soon, I was running for twenty minutes at a time. Sometimes I'd stop and walk a few minutes and then pick the pace back up, but I kept at it. I'd speed up when I could and slow down when I needed to. I started to look forward to my daily runs just for the "me time" they provided. I ran in my studio-monitor headphones. They were big and hot, but the music sounded great and that would charge me up for my run even more. I'd be locked into my favorite music and just zone out. This was a new way to experience life, like a third space that was different from any other type of exercise I was used to. I didn't need equipment; I didn't need a sparring partner. No commute, no gym, no dojo required. I didn't have to adjust my life around a class schedule. I could just wake up, put on my sneakers, and get to it first thing in the morning. The adrenaline, the music, the outdoors, the zone state of mind it put me in, I couldn't wait to feel that runner's high feeling again. I'd lay my shirt, shorts, socks, and shoes out the night before like we used to do before the first day of school. *Some me time to go train was all I wanted for Christmas.*

And then one day I finally hit the forty-five-minute mark and I remembered back to when Bones had first sparked my interest. I had come so far from barely being able to run ten solid minutes to being able to run a whole forty-five minutes without stopping. I felt fantastic. Soon I hit sixty minutes nonstop. Then I started tracking and measuring my time *and* distance. I was getting faster, too. I was getting my mileage and my speed up.

My runner's high was official.

Meeting Mr. Doubt

Running was my new passion. I was putting in roadwork anywhere from four to six days a week, sometimes twice a day. I went for shorter runs throughout the week and a longer run on the weekends. I had my sights set on earning a medal in Atlanta's world-famous Peachtree Road Race, which would be my first 10k.

I often trained at this dilapidated track not far from my house. A faded blue wooden sign bears the name "Quicksilver," the only thing that remains from its heyday. The track had been built for the '96 Olympics in Atlanta, then quickly abandoned and overgrown with tall grass patches and weeds once the Olympics came and left. Over the years since, the sun has baked, cracked, and warped the orange track so you have to really watch your step to avoid being tripped up by the folds and creases. Besides me, the only other usage the track got on a regular basis was by occasional walkers or groups of wild geese honking and foraging for insects and shitting all over the field. I'm referring to the goose shit, for clarity; there was a paved foot trail just off a bit in the bush for runners and walkers to go and discretely handle that kind of thing. 'Cause hey, shit happens.

I'd been consistently progressing, running three- and four-mile clips regularly over the last couple weeks, and was nearing my 10k race date. On this one particular day at Quicksilver my training goal was to run six miles nonstop, which would be the longest distance I'd run in one clip up to that point. One lap around Quicksilver was equal to a fourth of a mile so that meant I had to complete twenty-four laps to hit my six-mile PR (personal record) that day.

As I started making my first rounds there wasn't a cloud in the sky and the sun was beaming down with no mercy. I was listening to an audiobook—Hermann Hesse's *Siddartha*. I was already leaking sweat, dressed as I was in a hot-ass gray sweat suit and black combat boots. My logic for running in a sweat suit in the hot sun was for the psychological advantage I'd have on race day. Running in a tank, shorts, and sneakers would feel like light work compared to a sweat suit and boots. I was inspired by old footage of Muhammad Ali training at his Deer Lake Training Camp in combat boots. He would run in boots to add resistance to his roadwork, and so I jacked his technique and style. I had a method to the madness but that sun was not playing.

After I had completed about twelve laps that heat started to mess with me. There was a point where I was wringing sweat from my hoody like a dishrag.

And that's when I started seeing shit.

Squinting through the mirage-like heat waves rising up from the ground on the other side of the track, I saw what looked like an empty bench sitting on the inside perimeter. Only problem is there *ain't no benches* out there!

I finished another lap.

This time though, I saw what looked like a man sitting on the bench that wasn't there.

He wore a black fedora-style hat and a long black trench coat... giving off grim reaper–type vibes.

It was so hot I just assumed I was hallucinating. My mind was playing tricks on me. It was weird as hell.

But I kept seeing the image as if it were real.

The sun was brutal, and every step was feeling like jogging through quicksand. With multiple laps to go, my pace slowed down to barely a jog. I was doubting if I still had it in me to keep going. But just as I was about to give in to one of the excuses that was floating around in my head and cut my run short, I had a flash of insight about the mysterious man on the bench.

I had the sudden realization that I was projecting a personification of my own self-doubt. My insecurities were being shown to me in the form of an ominous-looking figure. When I realized this, things got even weirder. The man stood up and took off his coat, revealing a bright red-and-white tracksuit. I know it sounds crazy, but the mind works in mysterious ways.

I don't know why, but internally I instantly referred to the figure as "Mr. Doubt," and when I saw the tracksuit under his coat, I realized he was not a nemesis, but he was actually a coach in some strange way, or also like a scout there to keep me company. His doubtful scowl was not made with evil intent, it was a look of grit, a frown of determination. A screw face of fortitude. He wasn't there to frighten me but to help enlighten me.

The presence of this personified version of my own self-doubt reminded me that those doubts are just illusions, my mind playing tricks on me. I was inspired to be aware that when I'm feeling doubtful, I can embody the spirit of that mean mug on Mr. Doubt's face and turn that frown into fuel.

I kept going on that track feeling energized on the spirit level. Something inside assured me that from now on, Mr. Doubt will always be nearby on the sidelines seeing if I'm going to quit and give up or grit it out and keep going. He wasn't a grim reaper; he was a good teacher!

I hit my PR of six miles that day and ran an extra lap to celebrate what I had realized: doubts are not there to scare you into quitting, they are there to trigger and remind you of the spiritual determination you have inside you to endure and persevere. We overcome our doubts by realizing they are not real and stepping into our own magic. Like Marcus Garvey said, "If you haven't confidence in self, you are twice defeated in the race of life."

As time went on, I stayed ten toes down on my running regimen, logging literally hundreds of miles in my journal. As I toured around the world with dead prez, my training runs kept me focused and disciplined. In almost every city we rocked, beforehand I googled local routes, trails, and gyms with treadmills to get my roadwork in. I ran in Australia, Germany, Denmark, all over the US, South America. Every city I put in some roadwork. I medaled for 10Ks, and then half-marathons.

Then in 2012, I set my sights on what I believed at the time to be the black belt of distance running, the marathon: completing 26.2 miles nonstop.

I trained for almost a year for that thing—all around the city, on the road with dead prez, and even when we visited Chile, I banged out an epic high-altitude eighteen-mile run before the show that night. I almost passed out, but I made it. I had come a long way literally and figuratively. Back in Atlanta with just a couple weeks to go, I went to several sessions with our family doctor Dr. Wu, an award-winning acupuncturist and traditional Chinese herbalist, to charge my chi up for the upcoming race. My training regimen was relentless, and when October finally rolled around, I was charged and ready to get it!

AN EDUCATION ON RUNNING

I listened to tons of hours of audiobooks *about running* while running, too—from Cristopher McDougalls' *Born to Run*, to great reads by Rich Roll, a few of Dean Karnazes' books, *Chi-Running* by Danny Dreyer, Lopez Lomong's *Running for My Life*, *More Fire: How to Run the Kenyan Way* by Toby Tanser, Haile Gebrselassie's biography, *The Greatest*, written by Jim Denison, and so many more.

Learning about African and indigenous running traditions really inspired me. I realized that this running shit literally runs in our blood.

Atlanta Marathon Race Day

I woke up around 4:00 a.m., showered, meditated, and dressed in all black. I wanted to feel like Tyson stepping into the ring. I hydrated with water and coconut water and had a light breakfast: gluten-free peanut-butter toast and honeydew melon. My boy Dave Dread is a guy who loves adventure as a cyclist and a videographer and he had agreed to fly down from Washington, DC, ride his bike alongside me, and film the whole thing. That's a trouper, right?

So, we packed up his bike and camera gear, hopped in my Jeep, and made our way to the starting line downtown in Atlantic Station.

At about 6:00 a.m., still in the dark of the dawn, the cracking sound of the race starter's gun ricocheted in the air and, along with hundreds of other eager runners, with Dread following on his bike on the sidelines, I stepped into the mission I had been training for all year long.

It was go time.

The muted orange sky from the rising sun was spectacular as we runners made our way on the orange-coned route through the first stretches of our twenty-six-mile journey.

Miles one through six were light work, nice easy pace, passing by scores of spectators who were cheering us on with homemade signs and lighthearted motivational messages:

"You run better than the government."

"May the course be with you."

"Smile! Remember you paid to do this."

"Your feet hurt because you are kicking so much butt!"

I really appreciated all the creativity and thoughtfulness of all these folks who had come out so early and taken time out of their days to encourage us on our marathon journey.

One thing that stands out about the Atlanta Marathon course is the hills. There are no flat areas. It's just hill after hill after hill. I started to feel a slight touch of fatigue in my legs around mile six but it was no biggie. I steadied my breathing, in and out through the nose, as I'd learned to do hundreds of miles prior on my training runs. Dread would disappear and reappear as he found the best ways to film and keep up without obstructing the other runners on the course.

There was this one guy in the race, a tall, stoic-looking indigenous man with a red headband and tree trunk–looking legs. He caught my attention when I passed him by because of his laser-focused gaze and disposition...and he was not running, he was power walking! His pace was steady, intense, and relentless.

I had my earbuds in, bumping a playlist I curated with several hours of my favorite music, but there was so much fanfare and music bumping on the loudspeakers set up at different junctures along the course, it was hard to hear my own earbuds. I had made my marathon playlist to keep myself motivated, but what can you do? So, whenever I couldn't hear my own music in my earbuds I just flowed with the vibes in the moment as they were. One foot in front of the other.

Around mile twelve or so I was starting to feel the burn a little from those steep Atlanta hills, but I leaned into composer Bill Conti's "Gonna Fly Now" and "Going the Distance" and those tunes helped me to keep pushing forward. I probably played those joints like fifty times in a row.

Two hours passed, then three hours, and I was still running, not stopping. I didn't even stop for water. I would just grab a paper cup full as I passed by the volunteer stands, chug it in stride, and toss it to the side while I kept moving forward. Every now and then I'd look over and remember Dave was following on his bike with his camera catching the action, mile by mile.

What was super weird was that somehow, every so often, the indigenous brother who was power walking the whole race would appear out of nowhere, steady stomping through relentlessly. I'd be like, *I thought I passed him*? But somehow, he kept popping up, walking like a warrior; it was weird but his presence was inspiring. He was moving as fast and faster than many of us who were running. There's fast and then there's *steadfast,* and that's what he embodied. One step at a time, all the way.

By the time I was around mile twenty or so I started to hit that wall, where it seems like you just ain't got no more to give. With each step, it felt like my legs were being grabbed and held down by giant muscular arms reaching out of the asphalt. My spine was burning and no matter how much I wanted to push faster, it was all I could do to barely keep up the snail-like trot I was managing. But I kept going, one foot in front of the other.

The last stretch of the Atlanta Marathon, around the twenty-fourth mile marker, was a winding set of hills. I'd been running for almost four hours at this point and was beyond physically exhausted; it was all mental from here on out.

Mr. Doubt was pacing through the crowd on the sidelines, grilling me with that look on his face like a disappointed drill sergeant about to bite my head off. "Stop pussyfooting around," I imagined him saying. "Get this shit over with."

And then, finally, like a light at the end of a long, dark tunnel, I saw the finish line in sight and I got a boost of energy. The cheering from the sidelines intensified the sweetness of being steps away from accomplishing one of the toughest things I had ever set out to do.

With sweat dripping down my neck and pride fueling my last few steps, I made it back into Atlantic Station where it had all begun for me four hours earlier. I crossed the finish line at about four hours and some change, collapsing into a silver warming cape that one of the volunteers handed me as another put my medal over my neck.

That's done.

Well, almost.

The Marathon Continues

I'd just run 26.2 miles nonstop, but for me my day had just begun. The marathon was just breakfast. I couldn't quit my day job. I had a dead prez show scheduled that same night across the country in California.

With wobbly legs, I hobbled back to the Jeep with my buddy Dread, who, mind you, had also just skillfully filmed my run while cycling the whole marathon. Dread came through, yo!

I hit the crib, showered, and hugged my family who celebrated with me for a few quick moments. I ate a slice of homemade vegan sweet potato pie that my mom had brought over, and then I grabbed my bag and Afya took me straight to the airport to drop me off for my flight.

A piece of advice: if you can avoid it, never fly five hours across the country right after you just ran a marathon. It sucks. Sitting on that plane, my long-ass legs felt like sardines in a can. I was tired as shit and wanted to just pass out, but I had to keep waking up to stretch. Also, I didn't have a direct flight to LA—we had a layover in

Denver for a few hours. And then my connecting flight was delayed. So, by the time I finally arrived at LAX I had just enough time to check in at my hotel, freshen up for the stage, and then take off for the venue.

We dashed from the hotel through traffic over to the intimate Boar Cross'n venue in Carlsbad, arriving just in the nick of time. Rocking my white long-sleeve marathon finisher shirt with my medal swinging from my neck like a fat dookie rope, I burst in the front door of the spot, bopped through the crowd like 2Pac in a courtroom, and hopped onstage just as my dead prez comrades M-1 and DJ mikeflo were starting the intro! The crowd erupted as M-1 announced my entrance and congratulated me for coming straight from the marathon to the stage!

And we ripped that shit down that night.

In 2015, I became certified as a long-distance running coach by the RRCA (Road Runners Club of America) in Savannah, Georgia. Since then, I've been developing my own holistic coaching approach to running, incorporating inspiration from indigenous cultures, coaching myself, friends, and family, doing mindful running workshops, and of course still running and loving every step of the journey.

Going the distance is not really about how far you go or how fast you go, it's about being able to keep going. I found a path in running that has gotten me in the best shape of my life and taught me so much about the value of a steadfast attitude on my journey. It's just like the hip-hop mantra that has echoed from the earliest days—*and ya don't stop, keep on!* I'm so glad I followed up on Bones's challenge and started running. I never got my abs chiseled quite like his, but I found my fitness and something I value so much more—I realized I appreciate the dedication it brought to my life. I *enjoy* the discipline, and I discovered that I had the determination that allowed me to go the distance.

MOVEMENT IS LIFE, BREATH IS LIFE

The approach to exercise in the Western world is largely about the external body: the muscles, strength, competitive performance. But in many Eastern cultures, exercise is approached from a more internal angle. Inner vitality and physical health are more important than competitive dominance; this is cultivated through developing a deep mind-breath-body connection.

Hot Yoga

Yoga is a perfect example of an Eastern-style physical practice that is rooted in creating vitality from the inside out.

During one of our zillion convos on tour, my comrade and dead prez DJ mikeflo and I were trading stories in the back of a tour bus somewhere on the back roads of Europe. Flo told me about how he beat cancer and how liberating it was to be cancer free. He explained how having the cancer removed from his shoulder was a relief; it allowed him to open up to life in a more grateful and passionate way and it made him super focused on living in the now, prioritizing his self-care, mental health, and joy. He said he had been taking hot yoga classes and he thought I'd love it, too.

And he was right, I loved it!

Hot yoga classes are always a challenging and fulfilling treat. My first taste of hot yoga was a ninety-minute Bikram yoga practice; this consists of a series of medium-to-advanced standing and stretching postures in a room that feels like a cross between a steam room, sauna, sweat lodge, and a rainforest all in one. It's hot!

The intensity of the poses and the heat are designed to raise your heart rate, strengthen, relax, and lengthen your muscles, and detox your body through sweating. The intensity of the workout and the hot temperature ain't no joke. It's important to be well hydrated, and until you get used to it, you might feel light-headed or dizzy. There are people who are incredibly strong and flexible who do hot yoga and make it seem easy. Not me—I be in that bitch wobbling and taking mad breaks and sitting out whole sections of the routine when I need to, slurping my water bottle like a man stumbling into a desert oasis.

You'd think with all this going on it would be a miserable experience, but it's the opposite. At the end of class, you feel amazing. It's challenging but there's a method to the madness. There's something deeply therapeutic about how the class uses intensity to help you soften and relax. It's the same idea as the sweat lodge many indigenous cultures participate in to purge hearts, minds, spirits, and bodies in the heat; release toxins; and raise vibrations.

If we could see the intense experiences of our lives that inevitably come through the metaphorical lens of a hot yoga class or a sweat lodge, we could learn to appreciate the burn in a more meaningful way as a reminder to soften and relax instead of letting it make us cold. We can allow it to stretch and expand our inner peace through the chaos. When you are laying on that yoga mat after enduring the fire of a hot yoga experience and the instructor finally announces the final resting pose, Savasana, and you are lying there in corpse pose, and they crack open a door to start letting the cool air filter back in, you on your own little yoga mat island in an oasis of sweat, dripping in humble surrender, there's nothing like it. You start to feel the cool breeze ease back into the room and whisper over your body and the teacher comes by and places a cool lavender-scented towel on your forehead. That moment right there of deep, deep peace and relaxation makes it all worth it.

You'll be glad you namastayed.

Vitality: Breath is Life

The shape of the nose is like a pyramid
for those that know, it's a power grid
—Stic, "Qi Gong" Workout II

Pranayama is the science of breath in the yogic tradition. *Prana* means life-force energy (breath), *yama* means regulation. So, pranayama is a method of regulating the breath for greater vitality.

How long can you hold your breath? Let's do a drill right now and see.

Take a deep inhale and hold your breath. Slowly count down from sixty in your mind.

How'd you do?

If you held your breath for the whole minute, that's awesome. If you didn't make it all the way, that's fine, too. If you think you could have held your breath a lot longer than a minute, what would you wager your absolute max would be? Two minutes? Three? Maybe even five minutes if you absolutely had to? In 2021, the Guinness World Record holder was an incredible iron-lunged dude from Croatia named Budimir Šobat who fucking held his breath for twenty-four minutes and 37.36 seconds! That's almost as long as a whole sitcom episode (without the commercials).

The body's life force—prana, or chi—is carried into the body by oxygen, water, and food. This is why drinking lots of water, eating nourishing foods, and practicing breathing techniques are fundamental to all the ancient sciences of health and vitality. But dig this: you can go some weeks without food. You can go several days without water. But you can only go a couple of minutes without breathing. What does that tell you about how important breathing is?

Breath work is a vital category of exercise that is often overlooked and underappreciated. The more skillfully we breathe, the more vital energy we have for our lives.

Hertz So Good

Like yogis have done since ancient times, modern scientists have begun to examine the breath, exploring all that it can stimulate, regulate, and support in the body. The breath is connected with what the heart is doing, as well as the nervous system, the brain, blood, and all the organs and functions in the body. All these operations have their own frequencies and certain breathing techniques establish resonance with these internal functions.

When we slow our breathing to about six breaths per minute—that's about one inhale and exhale every ten seconds—that frequency translates to about a tenth of a hertz. Tiny, microscopic fluctuations in blood pressure create vibrations known as Mayer waves throughout our cardiovascular system that oscillate at that same frequency of 0.1 hertz.

That's also the frequency that's been studied and observed in the brains of people practicing Zen meditation, yoga mantras, and even some prayer rituals. When we inhale and exhale at the rate of around six breaths per minute it creates a calm resonance effect.

Breath work also helps us to better flow in our physical movements, concentrate our power, and focus it—like when we are lifting weights—and also improve our recovery time in between physical workouts. There are many studies that demonstrate the long list of benefits of breath training.

Here are four basic breathing practices to explore and add to your regimen.

Nose Breathing

What it is: The basic practice of breathing in and out through the nose. As newborns, we naturally breathe in and out through our noses. It's a survival design so we can breathe and suckle at the same time without choking.

What it do: Contrary to what you might think when you see people working out huffing and puffing with their mouths wide open gasping for air, nose breathing is actually the most efficient and advantageous way to breathe during exercise and in general. Nose breathing helps the lungs and heart work more efficiently during long-distance running and the controlled focus while engaging in dynamic activity helps you to enter into the zone state. Generally, nose breathing also helps filter out dust and allergens, boost oxygen uptake, increases nitric oxide in the body (that's a good thing), and humidifies the air we breathe in.

How to do it: Simple. Breathe with your mouth closed, in and out through the nose only.

Alternate Nostril Breathing

What it is: Alternate Nostril Breathing (ANB) is a **vitality** practice of breathing through alternate nostrils, one side at a time.

What it do: ANB helps clear out the nasal passageways, improving oxygen flow, and helps bring balance to the nervous system, slows your heart rate, and lowers blood pressure, all while destressing and soothing the mind.

How to do it: Breathe easy, gentle, and slow. Use your right thumb to block one nostril at a time.

1. Start with your RIGHT thumb blocking your RIGHT nostril.
2. With the right nostril covered, EXHALE slowly and deeply through your LEFT nostril.
3. Next cover your LEFT nostril and INHALE deeply and slowly in through your RIGHT nostril.
4. Next, KEEPING THE LEFT NOSTRIL COVERED, exhale through your right nostril.
5. Next, cover your right nostril with your thumb again but this time INHALE from your left nostril.
6. Repeat the full process for five to ten minutes.

Deep Belly Breathing

What it is: Deep belly breathing is a vitality practice, in which you expand and contract the belly (actually the diaphragm) with each in and out breath.

What it do: Deep belly breathing helps to slow your breathing so you can catch your breath and use less energy to breathe. It also helps get more oxygen into your lungs and calms you down so you can better control your breath.

How to do it: You'll be breathing in through the nose and out through the mouth.

1. Put your hands on your belly.
2. Close your mouth and take a slow, deep breath in through your nose. When you breathe in, you want your belly to fill with air and get bigger like a balloon.
3. For the exhale, blow all of the air out slowly and

gently through pursed lips like you were blowing bubbles.

4. Continue to breathe in through your nose and out through your mouth in this way. Practice for five to ten minutes.

*Note: You can also practice deep belly breathing and nose breathing together.

Box Breathing

What it is: Box breathing is a super simple tactical breathing technique used by the Navy SEALs, based on the "box-like" structure of the four equal parts.

What it do: Box breathing helps you regain calm and control of your thoughts when under stress.

How to do it:

1. Inhale for four seconds
2. Hold your lungs full for four seconds
3. Exhale for four seconds
4. Hold your lungs empty for four seconds

Repeat as many times as needed.

Movement Is Medicinal

Through the many different physical disciplines I've practiced over the years, I've gained so much more than physical benefits. I've become more self-aware and been able to tap into insights and higher perspectives for living that only come from putting in that work. Working out is a way I tap into my spirituality. A run is a prayer. A session of calisthenics is a church service. Sweat pouring out of my pores is libation. If I could blast it on billboards around the world, what I would say about exercise is: the physical *is spiritual*.

That's my training mindset out on that road putting in them miles, or on that bench, or on that yoga mat. My higher self, higher power, and higher purpose are in alignment. I love the runner's high I get when I settle and surrender into a long-distance run. It's a stress release. When I'm physically active, whether it be cardio, calisthenics, self-defense, or even just a country forest walk, I feel more relaxed and at peace. I love that muscle pump and soreness you get the day or so after you bang out a gang of push-ups or dumbbell reps. Insights and creative ideas flow so much better when I'm training on a consistent basis. I feel my best. I ain't competing with nobody else. My training is an investment in my well-being. It helps provide the strength, flexibility, endurance, and vitality for the life I wanna live. Here are some key takeaways for finding your fitness, things to be aware of, and what you might expect to experience on your journey.

DECIDE TO RIDE. Make a decision to make fitness a standard in your life. Get enthusiastic about moving your body on a regular basis doing something you enjoy. When you decide to ride, you're filled with motivation and excitement about fitness and exercise. Ride that wave.

DOUBT YOUR DOUBT. After the first rush of excitement, when you start to get to work, many times self-doubt enters the mind. It can either crush your momentum or it can make you stronger but it's gonna be a part of the process. How bad do you want this? Believe in the determination in your heart more than the doubts in your head. What powers self-confidence is your perspective. You can choose the perspective of doubt, focusing on what you feel you can't do, or you can choose a perspective of confidence and focus on what you can and will do. Your focus and perspective allow you to accomplish whatever you set your mind on. It might not always come easy, but each effort builds more self-confidence and that confidence carries over into the rest of your life.

NEW NORMAL. When you find your fitness, you see yourself in a whole new light. You embody this shit. You are a runner. You are a yogi. You are a cyclist. You now identify yourself as a fit and healthy person because of the consistency and results that have become a part of your life. You are the kind of person that prioritizes health and well-being and you've developed the discipline to walk the walk until it's become your new normal. Your discipline even inspires others around you.

KEEP RAISING THE BAR. Fitness is a lifelong process. It's not a destination, it's a never-ending journey. That's why you damn sure need to be enjoying the discipline on the way. When you've earned your own self-respect by staying on your regimen, nobody can take that from you. Keep elevating, keep challenging yourself, keep growing, keep winning! Stic to it!

Enjoy the Discipline

Bring an attitude of play to your fitness game.

Have you ever farted in yoga class or let one go at the gym? C'mon, just between me and you. No one will ever know but us. I know I've definitely let 'em go and sat there on my yoga mat with an innocent look on my face like "Ooh my, something *namastanks.*"

Like it wasn't my ass.

Seriously though, having fun in fitness (and in life) is *fun*damental. It's okay to lighten up even if it means lighting it up.

Okay, let's get serious for real here.

When we exercise with an *"I don't wanna be doing this shit"* attitude, it feels more like a chore than anything else, right? But when we lighten our attitude and approach it the way we might approach a game, that same amount of work becomes a form of play.

I was out for a run one day, hitting some challenging hills on one of my usual neighborhood routes, and I had this interesting realization: *I really like this shit.*

Now don't get me wrong. I'm not saying that those hills weren't kicking my ass, 'cause they were. I don't want you to mistake what I'm saying as this shit is easy.

But what I've realized is I actually like putting myself through these challenges. It gives me a sense of pride. My ability to appreciate and enjoy discipline is one of the things I like most about myself. It's so affirming to know I could be laying my ass up eating chips and drinking root beers growing a belly and not giving a fuck (which I sometimes also feel too) but instead I actually get a kick out of breaking a sweat, feeling the burn, investing in my wellness, and feeling accomplished when I'm done. The comfort zone feeling is cool, but that power zone feeling is amazing.

I'm not out here trying to be the fastest or the strongest or some super competitive athlete that's aiming to conquer the world of sport. I just actually enjoy the discipline of the training and how it invigorates my life. The lazy, lackadaisy comfort zone is a nice place to visit but I don't wanna live there 24-7. I like living in my *power* zone. There's nothing like a blood-pumping workout to make you feel more powerful, energized, and alive!

Some of us may think that using all our precious time watching TV, living vicariously through actors playing out the same old drama after drama, is the best use of our free time, but I just don't think that all this wonderful breath, bone, blood, and muscle that we are blessed with were meant to be squandered in our beds or on our couches glued to the TV screen all the time.

Change my mind! I'll wait!

The amount of time people spend watching TV is staggering. According to the market-research firm Nielsen, the average American household watches six to eight hours of television *a day*. That's a whole night of sleep's worth of TV! TV is a cool option to have. I ain't picking on TV, or TV watchers; it's an engaging form of entertainment and with all the content providers available, there's a wider range of things to watch that are of substance than ever before. But even still, active living opens the door for so much more joy and fulfillment in our lives than TV ever will. The TV show can wait, but life ain't gonna wait for nobody. If we get too comfortable, we start getting too soft and we start thinking shit is sweet out here a little too much.

The Bittersweet Science

Sister Kutchie, a Rasta herbalist and apothecary owner in my old neighborhood in Crown Heights, Brooklyn, would always say, "We need the bitters!" The "bitters" are healing root tinctures that might make you put on the ugly face when you swallow them but they're super good for your internal health and vitality. After a bit of adjustment, my taste buds stopped acting like li'l bitches and I learned to really enjoy her roots drinks and tonics.

It's so easy to enjoy the sweets of life but enjoying the bitter and the sweet and the sour and the tart and the salty and spicy and the pungent things of life makes for a well-rounded palate. Enjoying the discipline means being okay with making room in your comfort zone for healthy challenges. It means expanding your comfort zone to include things that exercise more of you. It's developing an *acquired* taste and appreciation for the uncomfortable things that empower us. We need the bitters.

No matter how young or old you are, challenging play is beneficial for the spirit. When we have a joyful connection to the exercise activities in our lives it can sometimes even make the effort feel almost effortless. I can see this principle at work easily with kids—if I ask my youngest son Kosi if he wants to go on a long-distance run with me, he more often than not will be like, "Nope, see you later Baba!" Once in a blue moon he'll tolerate it to spend some time with his dad, but the attitude is more, "I don't like it but I'm doing it," than anything else. But if I say, "Kosi! The zombies are chasing us!" and take off running, this little dude will leap into action! As long as he feels like we're *playing,* he is happy and motivated; the "exercise" takes care of itself because he enjoys it.

That simple fatherhood finesse is rooted in human psychology.

The reality of human behavior is that people are much more likely to do things that they enjoy. Duh, right? But it takes discipline to work out consistently, and that's just the facts. Most people like to play games more than they actually like to exercise. But here's the flip—creatively "psyching yourself up" and bringing an attitude of play to your exercise activities can help you find more joy in them. Experts say you don't need much. Just three hours a week is a decent minimum investment. But when you have lots of ways to make it fun, you'll be watching the clock less and enjoying the activities more!

Finding fitness that sticks and enjoying the discipline are all about striking a balance between purpose, process, and play.

- Purpose is your why: what makes the activity meaningful to you.
- Process is your how: the specific activity you're engaging in and how functional, practical, accessible, and doable it is for you.
- Play is the joy movement brings out of you and the fun attitude you bring to it. You like it, even if it's challenging, and you're enjoying yourself.

When these three elements are fulfilled, you'll definitely wanna keep coming back for more, so, here's a jewel to try and remember: in a challenging situation, always ask yourself: *What would make this more fun?*

You might not be able to create the ideal scenario every single time, but you can a lot of times. There are many great ways to bring more joy into your fitness training:

Add your favorite music—if you don't already, use your favorite tunes to motivate you. Every so often make a new playlist. I have different playlists curated around themes that inspire me and different types of workouts. My fit-hop albums *The Workout* and *Workout II* stay in constant rotation too because the lyrics are like affirmations for the healthy values I strive to live by.

Upgrade your location: in Chapter 3 we talked about switching up your routine. If you always train in the same location, it's good to break up the monotony. If you're always in the gym, get some action in the park. If you always run in your neighborhood, why not explore other parts of your city from time to time? A getaway ain't gotta be far away.

Enter a race: Nothing like a race day to look forward to and get excited about. Races help us tap into the electricity and adrenaline of competition and the medal you get at the end is a great keepsake to remind you of the fun and the accomplishment.

Accept a challenge: There are always new fitness challenges floating around on social media that you can tap into for inspiration. Follow various fitness accounts on the 'gram and you will be inundated with challenges to choose from. While you're at it, make sure @rbg-fitclub is one of them!

Take a class: If being around others motivates you to work out, then fitness classes are going to work great for you. Cycling, yoga, martial arts, Pilates, water aerobics...there are so many options to choose from! You may meet some new lifelong friends in the process.

Add rituals: Maybe grabbing a smoothie after your session could be your regular thing. Maybe a certain essential oil puts you in the zone. The little things we repeat, even if only symbolic, create a sense of familiarity in our practice that we can look forward to.

Make it up as you go: Freestyle is underrated. Just move. Do whatever. Shadow box, drop and do some push-ups, run sprints, stretch, dance. Ain't no rules to this shit. Give yourself permission to just enjoy breaking a sweat in whatever creative way that comes to you in the moment.

Get technical: Sometimes I like to focus in on one technique and just drill it over and over for a workout. Bruce Lee once said, "I fear not the man who has practiced ten thousand kicks once, but I fear the man who has practiced one kick ten thousand times." Zeroing in on a technique you want to improve is a fun way to give your practice a laser focus.

Role-play: Maybe the workouts that Michael B. Jordan did for his role in *Creed* would be fun to try on for size? Maybe Will Smith's *I Am Legend* pull-up regimen would be something interesting to explore? Actors have some incredible regimens that get them in shape for their roles. Get your Google on and become an action hero for a day!

Record yourself: In this generation of the selfie, it's never been easier to make a video of yourself working out. Recording and posting snippets of your workouts is a great way to make your training fun and motivate others.

Reward yourself: Reward goals can help you get it done! Give yourself a treat day on the weekend. Looking forward to buying yourself a new book or a fresh pair of sneakers if you hit a mileage goal works wonders for keeping you accountable and motivated.

Conduct an experiment: Get curious! When I wanted to gain twenty pounds on a plant-based diet, I conducted an experiment with Afya and my trainer to see if it was possible, and we self-published the results of our experience in the book *Eat Plants Lift Iron*. It was so challenging and fun.

Make it a service: Volunteer to help a friend move, ride your bike to the store for someone, volunteer for a community garden. Sweating for a cause greater than yourself pays off in many wonderful ways.

WHAT'S UP, DOC?

There ain't no shame in checking in with a health professional you trust to make sure you have a green light to do strenuous activities if you have any medical issues that you feel concerned about. The point is not to destroy yourself but to enjoy yourself. Be holistic and intentional with your fitness practice, bring your heart and dedication to it, and have fun.

Less Is More

> I do not compete with the rest of the world. I compete
> only with myself, for my progress is my true victory.
> —*Sri Chinmoy*

Many of the mainstream, status-quo ideas about fitness come from the perspective of athletic competition: go hard or go home; no pain, no gain; be the best; win, win, win—you know the vibes. But that's only one of many perspectives on approaching an active lifestyle. You don't have to be the heaviest lifter in the gym to get the benefits of weight lifting. You don't have to run the fastest or the farthest to get amazing benefits from running. You don't have to win every game to enjoy the sport. Competition demands bigger, stronger, faster, more, more, more. There is a time and a season for the no-pain-no-gain kind of approach, but that season is temporary and it definitely ain't sustainable or optimal for lifelong fitness.

My ego has taught me a lesson many times. I'd be out for a distance run, going at a comfortable enough pace for me to maintain, and along comes another runner moving much faster passing me by. Instantly my ego would start making comparisons and I'd find myself buying into the negative talk—telling myself how slow I was, that I must not be giving it my all—only to catch that same runner five minutes later, bent over catching their breath or walking or chugging on their water bottle.

They may have only been running one mile. They may be an Olympic athlete. The point is, who gives a fuck? You don't know what they are doing and comparing yourself to what they are doing takes the focus off what you are doing. The ego will fuck with you out there; stay mindful—run your race, your pace. This applies to life just as much as it does to running: don't compare yourself with others; everybody is on a different journey.

When it comes to doing fitness activities for health and wellness you don't have to always bring all that excessive, obsessive Olympic tryout anxiety to your practice. Sometimes less is actually more: the less stress we put on ourselves to perform better than somebody else, the more it can be beneficial, safe, restorative, and enjoyable. When your focus is health and well-being you can put less emphasis on competition and more emphasis on what's in the best interest of your vitality and longevity. Sometimes you push it, sometimes you pull it back a bit. Well-being is more a marathon than a spirit.

Exercising the four pillars—strength, flexibility, endurance, and vitality—has been the bedrock of what I strive for in my fitness training on a physical, mental, and spiritual level for the last two decades. At any point of the year, I may be in a phase where I'm emphasizing one or more of the pillars and I'm always open to try new methods to mix it up.

GAME TIME

The following are some gamified exercise options organized loosely under each of the four pillar categories to consider adding to your regimen. Sample from this list, take what's useful, ignore what isn't for you, and add your own custom spin. You can make a circuit selection of two or more of them or use one of the suggested exercises as a one-off workout by itself. And again, always remember these two things: **The best exercise program is always the one you'll actually do, and your only real competition is yesterday's you.**

Strength

Get stronger with these gamified exercise approaches.

Pyramids

The pyramids of Egypt literally embody what it means to be *built to last*—a reminder that when work is done well it remains solid. That's the same intention behind pyramid-style work-outs, or as some people call them, "ladders." The ancient Egyptian or Kemetic term for pyramids is *per ankh*, meaning "*house of life.*" With this calisthenics system, we are actually building mathematical pyramids with the body—our "house of life."

Pyramids are used in sports training programs for every-thing from football to powerlifting. They're used in the military to help soldiers quickly develop high volumes of repetitions, and pyramid-style workouts have long been used by inmates behind the wall to stay strong and come home swole. In gyms and parks and hoods everywhere, cats are getting in amazing shape using pyramid workouts because they provide a simple, go-to routine to get a nice pump, develop strength, and chisel certain muscle groups. The approach is great for general main-tenance as well.

How to Build a Pyramid: If you're unfamiliar with the terms reps and sets, it's simple: rep is short for repetition. One push-up, one sit-up, etc., is one "rep." A set is a group of *consecutive* reps. Some people also call a set a "clip" or even a "round," interchangeably.

In classic calisthenics, for a pyramid you are going to do multiple sets of your chosen exercise. Let's use push-ups as an example.

First, decide the maximum number of reps you want to do in one set. That determines the number of sets you'll do as well. For example, if you decide to go for 10 push-ups, that also means you're going to be doing ten sets of push-ups. But you're not going to do ten reps each set. That's where the pyramid comes in.

The crux of the pyramid system is doing one less or one more rep per set as you go.

So, if you want to build your pyramid from the top down, you start with ten push-ups and remove one rep each set until you get to one push-up.

If you want to build your pyramid bottom up, start with one push-up and add one to each set until you get to ten. As an example:

DOWNWARD PYRAMID: Ten push-ups, rest, then nine push-ups, rest, then eight, seven, and so forth down to one.

UPWARD PYRAMID: One push-up, rest, then two, rest, then three, on up to ten.

The upward pyramid and the downward pyramid are challenging in different ways. If you start with low reps, the reps will of course increase as you go. If you start off with higher reps, there are fewer and fewer reps to do as you go. Experiment with each way. And if you are feeling gangsta enough to do both in one workout session UP and DOWN, like a one-to-ten then ten-to-one flow back-to-back, you've got a built-in warm-up, max-out, and cooldown all rolled into one complete package.

Depending on your fitness level, I'd suggest starting anywhere from five to ten or fifteen sets max, but it's up to you. If you choose a number and can't quite make it through all the sets, it means two great things: one, you got a killer workout, and two, you've identified a benchmark to measure your future progress by.

Pyramids take the guesswork out of choosing a workout to do. All you have to do is choose your exercise and pick a target number of sets, decide if you wanna build it up, down, or both, and get to it!

I love doing pyramids with push-ups on sunny days in the park, on the pull-up bar I installed in our kitchen entryway, or just grabbing my earbuds and dumbbells from the side of the bed and getting in a quick morning pump or evening burn. I like to work on my kicking stamina with pyramids too—I'll do something like a fifteen to one on both legs. If you want more of a challenge you can try two or three or more rounds of a pyramid workout in one session. Go 'head with ya bad self!

You can even incorporate pyramids as a super set as a supplement to your standard weight lifting circuit: in between your regular sets, work in pyramid-style rounds of push-ups, squats, sit-ups, or whatever you want to throw in the mix for your goals. Also, since a DOWN pyramid progressively decreases your reps, it presents a perfect opportunity to add more weight each set.

Because of the built-in warm-ups and cooldowns in the pyramid system you might be surprised at the high amount of overall reps you'll actually be able to do. Pyramids are easy to customize and flexible for any fitness level. They're only limited by your imagination.

Rock The Bells Pyramid

Here's a pyramid-style workout for the iron, like dumbbells, barbells, and kettlebells. You'll do four sets of curls, or other lifts of your choice, with sets decreasing by five from twenty to five, resting between each.

You can even get creative and apply the pyramid concept

for running using distance or time as your variable for each set. For a time-based run pyramid, you might run for thirty minutes, rest, then run for twenty, rest, then run for ten. For a distance-based pyramid, you might run for three miles, rest, then do two miles, then one mile.

Fifty in the Clip

When you're mixing down songs in the recording studio there's a lot of downtime. You're sitting around for hours and hours listening, making tweaks, and giving feedback to the engineers as they work their magic for the final mix. In those sessions my homies and I would play a dice game to pass the time but instead of betting for money we played for push-ups. The purpose of the game was to help develop and maintain our crew standard of being able to do fifty push-ups in one set without stopping. Hence the name of the game, fifty in the clip. My boy Coach NYM or I would usually spark it off in the session. One of us would pull out the dice and start talking our let's-get-this-money talk, referring to exercise, and whoever else was around the studio that day, we'd peer pressure them into the action with us.

To walk around in the kind of shape where at any given point you could drop and do fifty push-ups nonstop, right on the spot, you have to do a lot of reps. When you get used to busting out clips of ten, twenty, twenty-five push-ups or more for round after round, hours at a time, the conditioning starts to quickly add up. We'd literally do nearly a thousand reps overnight some nights, sometimes even more. The more we played fifty in the clip the more conditioned we all got. If you ever dropped your flag on the ground, it was fifty in the clip on sight. If the homey wanted to test you he would challenge you to do fifty right there. We eventually even did a song about it called "50 in the Clip" on the dead prez album *RBG: Revolutionary but Gangsta*. It be so much fun and healthy competition, shit talking, and encouragement that you are way more in that game than you could be on your own. That teamwork makes everybody stronger. Iron sharpens iron.

How to play: All you need are three six-sided dice and at least two or more homies to play. We'd have anywhere from five to eight homies in a cypher at times.

Each game lasts ten rounds. Well, officially there's a ten-round minimum but we usually exceed that, and we even stopped counting rounds, you just bang out until you can't take any more. Up to you.

If you wanna quit before the agreed amount of rounds are done you have to pay a "let me out" tax of fifty push-ups.

A typical game would flow like this:

Each player makes their bet out loud for x number of push-ups.

Each round, everybody gets one roll of the three dice. Whoever throws the **highest point** wins the round and everybody else "pays" what they bet.

Scoring: The player throws all three dice together. To score a point you have to throw at least two matching number dice. The third dice is your "point." After everybody takes a turn, the highest point wins the round.

Single points can be six, five, four, three, or two, but if your point is a one that's "crap out," and you automatically lose and must pay what you bet.

Trips: If all three dice are the same, that's called trips. That beats any single point. Trip points can be three ones, twos, threes, fours, or fives. The highest number wins. If you roll three sixes you automatically win and everybody has to "pay you" what they bet. If you roll a four-five-six, it beats everything, even six-six-six. Once everyone has rolled and paid what is owed, a new round starts.

In the event that the highest points for the round are a tie, those players' bets automatically double and they do a tie-breaker roll. The loser has to pay up double. If you keep rolling ties it keeps doubling for the tiebreaker roll.

Tabatas

Got four minutes? The tabata protocol is a form of high-intensity interval training (HIIT) that alternates short bursts of exercise where you go super hard followed by even shorter recovery periods, and the whole workout only lasts four minutes.

It was originally devised by the head coach of the Japanese speed skating team in the 1990s, but it was his assistant Izumi Tabata who analyzed the effectiveness of the training method and published his findings in 1996 in the *Medicine & Science in Sports & Exercise* journal and ended up stealing the spotlight and the namesake.

Tabata training increases both short-term explosive strength *and* long-term endurance. It also continues to burn fat for several hours after the workout is done.

A group study of people who did a four-minute tabata session five times per week showed more improvement than a control group who did one hour of steady training five times a week, over the course of six weeks. That means the cats that did tabatas, who only worked out twenty minutes a week, showed more improvements than the control group who worked out five hours a week!

How to do it: The protocol for tabatas is super easy. Warm up before you start with easy arm circles or a minute or so of jumping jacks—just something to get the blood pumping so you don't start out cold. Tabatas are INTENSE!

Once you feel warmed up and ready, you're going to choose an exercise and do twenty seconds of maximum effort with ten seconds of rest, repeated eight times for a total of four minutes.

That's it. The key is you gotta really go hard in the twenty-second parts, and then really chill for the ten seconds of recovery. It's helpful to download a good tabata timer app like Tabata Pro or Tabata Timer.

Another bonus of tabata training is that it can be done with all kinds of exercises. An indoor bike is how Dr. Tabata conducted his research, but you could use:

- A rowing machine
- Running sprints
- Burpees
- Squat jumps
- Jump rope
- Shadow boxing

Or anything else you like.

You can also switch up the exercises during the workout, to add some variety. You might do burpees for the first twenty seconds, then do shadow boxing or squats for the next twenty seconds, and so forth. Aim for three or four times per week maximum, but start off easy. Tabatas ain't no joke, fam.

Scale the workout to your level of fitness. Don't kill ya self with burpees if you ain't there yet. If a fast walk up a hill is going hard for you and that's what elevates your heart rate, do that! Get stronger one step at a time.

Dragon Sit-Ups

> My strength comes from the abdomen. It's the center of gravity and the source of real power. The proper way of doing sit-ups isn't just to go up and down, but to curl yourself up; to curl your back up, like rolling up a roll of paper.
>
> —Bruce Lee

Bruce Lee's version of the sit-up targeted the upper abdominals and intercostal muscles under the ribs. He did high repetitions to maximize the impact.

How to do it: You'll be doing four sets of twenty reps. Lie down, bend your knees slightly, then roll your torso upward until your chest is pressed firmly against your knees. Hold this fully contracted position for one to two seconds, then return to the starting position.

As you rise up, touch your left elbow to your right knee, then on the next rep, touch your right elbow to the left knee.

Vitality

Cultivate your internal vitality with these breath, body, and mind exercises.

Blue Kidney Drill

According to traditional-Chinese-medicine theory, this qigong practice nourishes the kidney meridian—which functions like the battery of the body. When the kidneys are strong, nourished, and functioning well, vital energy increases throughout the body.

1. Make fists with both hands and place the knuckles of each on your lower back.
2. Inhale through the nose.
3. As you do, imagine a mist of blue light traveling into your kidneys.
4. As you exhale, say "Fuuuuuuuu!" or "Choooooo!" for the duration of your exhale.
5. Start by practicing for five to ten minutes, building up to one hour.
6. Add meditation music to set a Zen tone to your practice.

Bruce Lee Moments

Bruce Lee was great at making every moment count; he seamlessly integrated fitness training into all aspects of his life. He wouldn't just sit and watch TV, he'd lift dumbbells during the commercials. While he was reading or studying, he'd be simultaneously stretching or cycling on his exercise bike. Instead of parking close to his destination he'd park farther out to get more of a leg workout out of his errand. Instead of the elevator or escalator he'd take the stairs. He was always finding opportunities to make the most out of his day by squeezing in fitness in creative ways.

So, a Bruce Lee Moment is any time you squeeze more fitness activities into the regular moments of our lives in creative ways, like:

- Push-ups while pumping gas: You'll start to associate pumping gas with feeling a pump yourself. Just put a towel down because gas stations are grimy. Running in place while you fill up is another option if you don't wanna get your hands dirty.

- Walking or running while in phone meetings
- Light shadow boxing in the parking lot while waiting on takeout
- Meditating on a flight
- Practicing breathing exercises while commuting
- Getting off the bus earlier and walking farther to your destination
- Park farther away at the grocery store
- Stretch while watching your favorite show
- Take the stairs instead of the elevator

There are so many other ways to practice the art of making mundane moments into creative fitness opportunities. Every little bit adds up, so, the next time you have the opportunity to incorporate fitness into your life, ask yourself, What would Bruce Lee do?

He would make the moments count. And so can we!

Upside-Downs (Inversions)

Better for you than a shot of espresso, inversions can hit you with a boost of energy to start your day or give you an energy boost whenever you need one.

What it is: Inversions, or upside-downs, are a category of static exercises that place your head below your heart and hips, "inverting" your body from its regular upright position. Asanas like downward dogs, handstands, headstands, shoulder stands, putting your legs up on the wall, etc., are good examples.

What it do: Inversions help improve circulation, letting blood rush to your head and helping to lower blood pressure and heart rate. Inversions give your circulatory system a helping hand in moving blood around to all the places it has to travel, without having to fight gravity to do so. This gives your heart and circulatory system a nice rest. Upside-downs help the flow of your oxygenated blood get to the brain, upper organs, and the face easier. Improved circulation of the flow of blood and oxygen to your brain also helps with concentration and memory. Inversions also:

- ease venous return flow, helping deoxygenated blood travel back to your heart,
- help the lymphatic system process toxins, and
- positively impact the nervous system. Inversions engage the diaphragm, which activates the parasympathetic nervous system to calm the nerves.

How to do it: I'm giving you two easy upside-down poses to try, but you can research others and up your inversion game.

Inversion 1: Legs up the Wall

Lie on your back and scoot your butt up against a wall. Put both your legs up the surface of the wall, forming an L shape with your body. If your lower back and hamstrings are too tight, instead of leaning up against a wall, you can easily modify by using a chair or even the edge of your bed. With the chair or bed variation, you'll bend your legs at the knee to form a 90-degree angle and let your lower legs and feet just rest on top of the chair or bed.

For the wall version or the bed or chair variation, you can place a pillow under your head to make it more comfortable if you like. Feel free to use a folded blanket or two or a yoga block to raise your hips up more and see how that feels.

Start with anywhere from three to five minutes and work

your way up to fifteen minutes or whatever feels like enough for you.

Doing legs up the wall before bed is dope to give your feet and legs some extra relief; it'll help you feel more relaxed and ready for a good night's rest.

Inversion 2: Melting Heart Prayer

On your hands and knees, walk your hands forward and allow your chest to move down toward the floor. Try to bring your forehead or chin to the floor. If your chest can't reach the ground, use a yoga block or something similar. Keep your hips right above your knees and your hands shoulder-width apart, so that you're lightly arching your back with your butt up in the air and your arms stretched out in front of you, palms down. You can put a soft pillow or folded blanket underneath your knees to make it more comfortable. Your toes can either be tucked under, toenails facing the floor, or your toes can be flexed facing forward.

Once you're in the position, just relax there and let your breath flow in and out.

Come out of the pose by just gently sliding forward onto your stomach.

If you feel any pain, discomfort, or tingling, adjust your arms and hand positions. It ain't supposed to hurt—it should be relaxing.

Try to hold it for one to two minutes and work your way up to five minutes.

Resting Squat Hold

Starting in first grade, we're made to sit in a chair for hours a day, five days a week. If you're at a job that has you sitting all day, or if you're a creative on a computer for hours at a time, this is a great exercise to help counteract the stress on your lower back.

What it is: In this hold, you'll lower your body down from a standing position, until your legs are completely bent while keeping your back as straight as possible and your feet still flat on the ground.

What it do: The better your ability to squat, the healthier your spine, lower back, joints, and muscles will be.

How to do it: While keeping both of your feet flat on the floor, squat down as low as possible. Keep your knees pointed in the same direction as your toes, making sure your back is not hunched over but is as erect as possible.

Hold the squat for thirty seconds. Work your way up to one to three minutes.

You can make a ten-minute circuit out of it by doing five one-minute squats with one-minute rests in between each interval until you hit ten minutes.

DRESS FRESH + GEAR UP

As shallow as it may seem, dressing fly for your workout is actually quite effective. Putting on some fresh shit that you look and feel good in will help you enjoy your workout more every time. If those sunny yellow sneakers are going to inspire you to bang out your run with more pep in your step, by all means, buy them shits. That's a health investment!

If you like to stay up on the latest athletic tech gear and having the newest apps or gadgets to measure your activities is gonna motivate you to move more, by all means, indulge your toys, for the good of your health.

When it comes to clothes and gear, invest in quality not quantity. Of course, don't waste your bread on things you ain't gonna use, but if it's gonna help you move...rock it! Look good and feel good!

Endurance

Here are a few creative suggestions for incorporating endurance in your practice.

Sage Runs

A sage run is a ritual form of running that I created, *inspired* by indigenous (Native American) running cultures. These runs provide a ceremonial gateway as they use running as a form of intention, prayer, emotional healing, spiritual cleansing, or creative meditation, or in honor of a special occasion. Running while burning sage creates a sacred ceremonial atmosphere along your path and elevates your run as an offering toward your spiritual intention. It can be done solo or in groups, for celebrations, for mourning, for birthdays, for going-aways, for big decisions, to process strong emotions, for rites of passage, or just to express gratitude for life.

How to do it: Get a small bundle-stick of white sage. Determine the amount of time or distance for your run—it don't have to be nothing crazy. A sage run is not a purely physical fitness thing. It's symbolic. If you want to push yourself and go mad hard, fast, or far to intensify the spiritual vibration, by all means, do so. But there's nothing ineffective about keeping it light and easy. It's all about the intention and honoring that throughout the run.

Take a few deep breaths to just settle into a calm mind space. As you light the sage, which you will also be running with, speak some heartfelt words out loud expressing what the run is in honor of. For example, "This sage run is in honor of the birth of my unborn child, for their healthy arrival, and for my spouse to experience a natural, safe delivery." Blow into the burning sage and let the smoke billow up as a metaphor for your intention traveling out into the universe.

Begin the run holding the sage like a torch as it burns. Be careful not to burn yourself because the flakes and embers will fly off from time to time. Be especially mindful if you're running in the forest or on a trail. Keep the intention of your run in your heart and mind throughout the run. Visualize the outcome of your intention.

When you are done, close the ritual with any words or prayers or silence—whatever feels right to you—and make sure to fully extinguish the sage, safely.

Also: keep a lighter handy in case the sage goes out midrun. Try to keep it lit until the run is complete.

Three by Threes

I learned this super simple routine from the boxing gym. It's a pretty standard warm-up that gets the blood pumping and circulating right away. It's a great way to work on your cardio, footwork, coordination, and muscular tone all in one.

You can do this as soon as you wake up in the morning or any time you've got less than fifteen minutes to spare. All you need are a jump rope and a timer—there are some cool apps boxers use that allow you to set a timer for the active round and the resting round. For the rope, try a lightweight speed rope; you can take it with you anywhere and get a fantastic boxer's burn in between meetings or when you step away from your desk for a quick cardio break. Come back up in that bitch feeling like a champ.

How to do it: As the name implies, this one is pretty simple. Skip rope for a total of three three-minute rounds. Rest one minute between each round. The whole workout takes just twelve minutes.

Squat Life

Squats are one of the simplest yet most effective exercises that you can do. This marathon of squats will trigger lower-body muscle gains in size, strength, and tone, and boost your metabolism and burn a shit load of calories. This squat workout is beast mode for your legs.

The mission: complete one thousand squats in a day. You can do one thousand reps as a onetime challenge, or as a regular weekly, monthly, or seasonal treat.

There's an African proverb that goes, "How do you eat the head of a rat? Bit by bit." It might be disgusting, but it perfectly describes how to go about doing something hard—you break it down into bite-size pieces. So, here are three techniques to chew on as options for attacking this squat challenge:

ALL DAY. Do ten sets of one hundred squats spaced throughout your day. Choose this if you want to spread the work out over the course of the day so you can take breaks, but also give yourself a nice, energizing boost with each set.

BANG OUTS. Crank out fifty sets of twenty-five, or one hundred sets of ten, or however you need or want to break it down. Rest just enough to prepare for your next set. Choose this if you just wanna get the shit out the way and be done with it!

MINUTE TO WIN IT. Do fifteen to twenty squats per minute. Rest and repeat until you reach a total of one thousand. This is brutal but the bragging rights are yours for life.

You can also apply this to other movements:

One Thousand Kicks. You can choose a specific kick style you want to focus on—one thousand front, side, low, or high kicks—or you can mix it up and do several different kicks spread out over the thousand-rep challenge. Try your best to keep good form as you get exhausted. It ain't a race. Take your time and take small breaks when you need to. Other than that, the only rule is don't quit!

Two Hundred Pull-Ups. Earlier, I mentioned how Afya and I had to do this workout as an initiation into the ijala martial-arts class. It's grueling. It might even seem impossible. But the feeling of getting it done will teach you something about yourself that will last long after the pain has faded.

Easy work. Eat that rat.

Flexibility

To remain flexible, consistent stretching is a must. There's no getting around it. It's my least favorite exercise to do, so I have to continue to make extra effort to stay inspired and incorporate it in regular ways. Here are some ways I do it.

Around the Worlds

Around the World in a Day is an easy system for implementing more stretching into your days without having to give it much thought. By incorporating mini moments of stretching throughout the day, dedicating just a few minutes at a time, you can bang out twenty minutes of stretching over the course of twelve hours. It might not seem like much, but twenty minutes of stretching a day goes a long way.

How to do it: Split your day into four quadrants: morning, midday, evening, and bedtime.

What you'll do is coordinate these quadrants of your day

with specific areas of your body for short, focused stretching. For example:

- Morning: focus on the upper body with five minutes of simple upper-body stretching
- Midday: focus on your midsection (abs, lower back) for five minutes
- Evening: stretch out your hips for five minutes
- Bedtime: stretch your legs for five minutes

Five minutes here and there is easy to fit in and makes for some good breaks to keep your circulation flowing through the day. Doing this just a couple times a week is better than no stretching at all.

Hang Times

Hang times (also called dead hangs) stretch the shoulders, arms, and back, and decompress and stretch out the spine.

What it is: You simply hang from a pull-up bar.

What it do: Hang times are especially beneficial if you sit a lot for work or if your back muscles are tight and sore and you need to stretch them out. Hang times also strengthen the upper back, shoulders, core, forearms, grip strength, hands, and wrists. Dead hangs are a good first step to getting your body ready to do pull-ups, if you're new to them.

How to do it:

1. You'll need a pull-up bar.
2. Grip the bar with your palms facing away from you (overhand grip). Keep your arms shoulder-width apart.

3. Hang, keeping your arms straight. Don't bend them, just hang like a heavy bag, keep your breath flowing, and stay relaxed.

Hang for ten seconds to start and try two to three sets. Set a goal to work your way up to three sets of thirty-second hangs, or forty-five seconds to one minute if you like. As a variation, you can try an underhand grip with your palms facing toward you. Hang in there!

PUTTING THE FOUR PILLARS TOGETHER

Here are two easy ways to bring all the four pillars into your routine.

Four-Pillar Ten-Minute Charge Up

Jumping jacks for one minute
Push-ups for one minute
Squats for one minute
V-ups (jackknife sit-ups) for one minute
Plank for one minute
Finish with a five-minute meditation

Four-Pillar Power Hour

Choose à la carte:
Fifteen-minute cardio
Fifteen-minute calisthenics
Fifteen-minute stretching
Fifteen-minute breath work

PRINCIPLE 4

RESTORATION

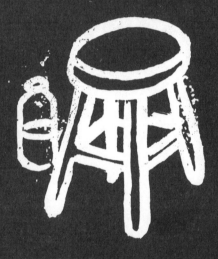

CHAPTER 12

The Wheel of Life

I can enjoy a hundred dollars in good health better than you can enjoy a million dollars in bad health.

—*Styles P*

L et me confess right off the bat: I'm a grind-aholic in recovery. I learned early coming up that if you don't work you don't eat and if you don't grind you don't shine. You know the codes: no struggle, no progress; no pain, no gain; no hustle, no harvest. I've been living by these mantras for decades. They got me through a lot. People who really know me always see me going hard in the paint, training, study-ing, handling multiple business projects 24-7, making music, touring, and I always got my hand in a new creative hustle. When I was maybe seventeen or so, one of my closest Ogs at the time hit me with the jewel that a man is supposed to be to his family what the sun is to the Earth. The sun is the provider. The sun don't chill, god. He taught me that our job as men, like the sun, is to provide our light and energy and warmth, 365 days a year, to make sure our Earth has what she needs to make the family thrive. And you also have to take into account the rest of the galaxy—your extended fam and homies that need you, too. Being the sun of your universe takes a lot of energy. A whole lot.

Sometimes it can feel like you're setting yourself on fire to keep other people warm. But to me, it's an honor to serve. I learned that value from my mom. She is one of the most selfless, giving, hardworking, and genuinely generous people you could ever meet. If you are homeless and you happen to meet my mom, you are going to eat good that day, and you just might—'cause she's done it a gang of times—get offered a room at her house while she helps you find your way. My mom stood on her feet for years doing hair in our kitchen to help put food in our mouths and taught me what it means to push through when you're tired to take care of your business and provide for those you love. She would always say, "*Baby, whatever you do in life make sure you love it, because when it get hard you have to being doing it out of love or it ain't gonna work.*"

When she and Pops divorced, my sense of manning up went through the roof. I felt a heavy responsibility to try to take care of her and everything and everybody I love. That's where my drive to go hard, make moves, and make shit happen comes from. Afya and my closest loved ones are always looking out for me and reminding me to take breaks and get some rest when they see I need it. It's spooky how easy mom dukes can see it man; you can't hide how you feel from mom dukes. I'll get off the road, then jump right into washing clothes or I'll be washing dishes and cleaning the kitchen all while strategizing my next moves in my mind and my mom will come over to visit and right away she'll be like, "Baby, you need to get you some rest." I be like, "You right, Mom. I will. I'm alright." But inside I'm like, "The grind don't stop 'cause the game don't wait."

The hustle in me has helped me man up and take care of business and take care of my family when I ain't had nothing else but my grind. When I left home and went to New York to chase my dreams of getting a record deal, it didn't happen overnight. It was cold and New York don't give a fuck about your dreams. You got to make 'em respect your dream with your hustle. And in chasing that dream, I was even homeless for a stretch, G. I know what it feels like to be at that lowest low—to have to ask a stranger for some spare change. To be hungry but have to wait on next month's food stamps just to be able to eat. I vowed to never be in that position again. I became a hunter. A hustler spirit ain't nothing but that primal instinct in us to go hunt and bring back the food. Every time I eat a meal, I take a moment and I give thanks. I don't take it for granted.

That "go hard and go get it" mentality has helped me create opportunities and make power moves that taking it easy all the time just ain't gonna do. I became addicted to the grind. I'm allergic to not putting in work. Sitting around and chilling too much be feeling like I'm wasting time and not being as productive as I could be. I rather be active, so I'm always plotting and planning and strategizing on getting to the bag. That just makes sense where I'm from. It's the same drive that helped me run twenty-six miles in a marathon; produce, write, and release my own albums; write books; start brands; produce films—and all type of other moves I make that require a lot of grind time to make happen. I want my family to have what they need and want. Being worried about where the next meal or the next mortgage payment or the next money is going to come from ain't the movement. It ain't 'cause I'm on some capitalist shit with it, it's just the water we swimming in. The game takes money to play. You ain't gotta like the game, you don't gotta love the water, you ain't gotta be selfish with the water neither, but as long as you in the water you either gonna swim or you gonna drown. Nobody ain't gonna make your goals happen for you. You got to go get 'em. And that mentality has served me well as a provider taking care of my family for the last two decades. But being a relentless go-getter can sometimes be a gift and a curse.

———

You know you're going way too hard when your hair starts falling out on you. I was in my midthirties and had been living in the A for a few years by then. I had a gang of shit going on at the time, as usual, and I was just feeling stressed to the max. My brother was still getting into one thing after another and still going back and forth to prison for years, and I was worried about him all the time. I was pissed because of how his choices affect my mom. I was away from my family a lot 'cause we were doing dead prez shows back-to-back. I was jumping on and off planes, living out of bags from hotel to hotel, and it was getting stressful dealing with all the different drama that be on the road. When I was off the road, I was working on music late nights in the studio or doing fifty million other things to stay on top of bills and expenses and shit like that, so even though I'd be home off the road at times, I still wasn't really getting no real rest. I was feeling irritable and overwhelmed, and I didn't really know what I could do about it. Like Jamaicans say *lotta ting agwon*.

I woke up one morning and was in the bathroom and looking at myself in the mirror. I could see bags under my eyes, and I was just looking run-down and tired as a motherfucker. I hadn't even had a haircut in a while.

Afya came in the bathroom and said, "Are you going bald?"

I was like "Bald? What you mean?"

She palmed the back of my head and started feeling around.

"Did you get nicked at the barbershop the last time you got a cut?" she asked. "It looks like you got a bald spot back here."

I got the small mirror off the counter to see the back of my head in the big mirror in our bathroom and I saw this bald spot about the size of a quarter.

"Yoooo! What the fuck? On top of everything I'm dealing with, now I'm going bald too?"

It turned out that bald spot was a condition called alopecia. When Afya and I did the knowledge, we learned that alopecia can come from all kinds of reasons, but in my case we both felt like it came from stress. That patch of missing hair was my body saying, "Bro you out of balance."

Afya got to doing her research on natural remedies like she always do, mixed together some herbs into a paste, and massaged it into my scalp on top of the bald spot with a Q-tip. Afya was sweet to me and tried to make me feel like it wasn't that bad and reassured me that it would heal up soon, and I appreciated her for being so loving and kind about it, but that shit was still embarrassing to me. I started wearing my black skully every day, even when I was just around the house.

Afya is also a holistic health counselor, and I had seen her work her helpful magic in many lives. I thought to myself, "Shit, I might benefit from some holistic counseling my damn self." I asked her if she could take me on as a client and put me on her schedule to help me deal with stress better. I felt like I really needed it.

"Okay, I got you," she said.

Reestablishing Balance

Our first session was at our crib at the dining-room table. She handed me a blue folder that said Khnum on it with a bunch of papers in it. She started explaining to me that holistic health counseling is a way to help people experience more healing, balance, and joy in all the different areas of their lives. Then she had me answer a lot of self-searching questions so I could zero in and really think about and pinpoint the main challenges I was having. The tool that she shared that impacted me the most, and one I've been using ever since, was a powerful exercise she learned in her studies at the Institute for Integrative Nutrition in NYC. It's called the wheel of life, and yo, it was a game changer!

The wheel of life is one of those things that after you get hip to it, you wonder how you were able to ever function without it. It's a super simple way to look at eight of the most important areas of your life as a whole. It gives you a clear visual picture of where your life is thriving and what areas could use a little more work. The categories are: health, fitness, work/career, joy, relationship, friendships, finance, and spirituality—all the big areas of life. It's crazy how before we even started the exercise, just seeing the list of eight categories helped immediately. It took what was seeming like a zillion chaotic things going on in my life all the time and simplified it all into eight clear areas to focus on. It was as if my mind were a messy desk and she just took all the clutter scattered all over it and organized it into neat folders.

To get into it, you rate your current level of satisfaction on a scale from one to ten by marking dots on a circular pie graph that's divided into the eight areas. For each area you place a dot based on how you feel. A dot closer to the center means you feel less satisfied in that area, a dot closer to the edge of the circle means you're more satisfied in that area. When you're finished making your dots in all eight categories, you draw a line from dot to dot to connect all the dots and you get a "shape." So, in theory, if you felt super satisfied in all eight areas and marked all your dots at the points indicating a ten, your shape would be a circle.

But say you felt like money is tight so you marked a dot at the three point for finances. Your relationship is going through it at the moment, so you marked a two. Let's say you've been at the gym a lot lately and you actually feel good about your fitness so you mark an eight. Now, if you were to connect *those* dots you won't have a nice, even circle shape. When I looked at the shape of mine that day it looked more like a raggedy star than a circle. The categories you rate highest show you the areas you're most thriving in. And that's super important when you stressed the fuck out, in the middle of all that, to be able to appreciate something that is actually working right. It's always something to be grateful for. And then those areas you rated lowest show you what to focus in on to balance your life more across the board.

Afya coached me through filling out the wheel of life exercise by asking me how satisfied I felt in each area, and I marked my answer numerically on the chart for each one. Then she went on to teach me how to understand my results. The aha moment was when I realized she was not solving my problem; she was removing what was in the way of me finding my own solution: all the overwhelming feelings I felt. I had been knocked off-balance by having too much going on and the wheel exercise gave me a visual POV to reestablish what balance could look like in the face of all I was dealing with.

That reset was a revelation. It felt like reestablishing my proper fighting stance for life. You know how in boxing or martial arts, when your hands are up, elbows down, your chin is tucked, your legs are bent a little bit, and you're on the balls of your feet, you can pivot? You're loose; you're balanced and ready for whatever. That's what the wheel exercise did for me. It recalibrated my balance. When life is kicking your ass and you're stressed, it's important to get back in your fighting stance, to realign and rebalance yourself. When you are stressed, it can feel like you are in the middle of a fight, getting beat up, like you're not keeping your hands up and you're tripping over your own feet and getting thrown off-balance. The refocus that the wheel exercise gives you is like a cornerman telling you how to pull yourself together and get your head back in the game so you can better deal with what's in front of you in the ring of life. We all get caught off guard, it's just about having the mindfulness to refresh and recenter.

That counseling session with Afya got me back in the fight. I saw where I was slipping the most was that I wasn't balancing my rest and relaxation time with my grind time. I didn't know how to be off and just actually relax. I do so many things I love to do professionally, but outside of that I didn't have no real hobbies. I was doing too much and going too hard all day, every day, and not respecting the balance, and that alopecia patch on the back of my head was trying to let me know it's time for a break. My body was saying, "You gots to chill."

I made a commitment to start respecting rest more and to intentionally create space for more relaxation in my schedule.

The Science of Sleep

Not too long after the counseling sessions with Afya, I was moving through an airport and I picked up a copy of *The Sleep Revolution*, the best-selling book written by Arianna Huffington, who founded the *Huffington Post*. It was perfect timing 'cause I wanted to pick up game on how to improve on rest in general, and I had seen reviews that said her book was thorough. And man, was it!

I was supposed to be resting on the damn flight, but I couldn't put it down. She drops gem after gem on how lack of rest affects every area of our lives. She touched on everything, from how hard it is at times to prioritize getting enough rest in the society we live in, where everything is on go-mode twenty-four hours a day, to how it still seems like it ain't enough hours in the day sometimes. I resonated with the way she spoke on how, when you do have time to relax, it's still tough to let yourself wind down and surrender to just chilling, and even just how hard it can be to fall asleep and stay asleep when we do try to get rest, because the mind is always racing all the time.

It's deep in the fabric of the culture of society. It's the capitalist way to just grind, grind, grind. It ain't just coffee beans at Starbucks that's getting ground up by the millions every day; this grind-'til-we-drop lifestyle is grinding people up just like them coffee beans. Shit, New York City prides itself as the city that never sleeps. Nas is famous for that classic bar he spit where he said, "I never sleep 'cause sleep is the cousin of death." That's the best advice when you take it to mean stay woke to the bullshit out here, stay hip to the games people play, and be sharp and aware. Yeah, don't ever sleep in that sense; but when you apply that "never sleep" shit to your grind, that's self-destruction in the making. You know what happens when you don't stop and you just keep going, burn, burn, burn, burning the midnight oil? You burn out. But when we can start to put things in perspective and start to balance all the doing and going with more relaxing and flowing in our lives, that's like the main thing that sets off the domino effect that feeds all the other areas of healthy living.

The science of what happens when we sleep and how it affects our lives is deep, yo. The more I learn about rest and relaxation, the more I respect it. When you clocking them zzz's, your organs and all the systems in the body slow down for repair and recovery from the day. Overnight, like clockwork, hormones flood your body—like your own inner night-shift crew of chemicals and functions that clock in on schedule and get busy. Your pineal gland produces melatonin (which helps you relax and feel sleepy). Your pituitary gland releases hormones that help the body to repair itself. Your food is getting digested, cells are getting healed and regenerated. If you've been banging out on the iron in the gym that's when the muscles get the time and chemicals they need to grow. Your memories get filed and organized and your subconscious sends you insights and messages through dreams. Without sleep, all these vital functions are disrupted and the compound effect shows up as less daily energy, weakening of the immune system, increased stress levels, and more.

To say sleep is necessary is an understatement. Sleep is the plug. Nah, better yet, sleep is the gold reserve that backs up the currency of energy we spend every day. It bankrolls how we invest our time. Sleep is kind of like the credit card of the body. You put charges on your sleep account by how you spend your energy and time every day and you pay the bill back every night when you get rest. Then waking up energized for your day, that's like having good credit. As long as you keep using your energy card and don't miss them sleep payments, you're establishing that good credit, and you can tell because you wake up on the right side of the bed, feeling energized in your life instead of drained and exhausted all the time. And just like a credit card works, as you keep up those rest and relaxation payments, your daily energy limit goes up. That's how you get that high credit score, where you feel like anything you need or want to do you have the energy available in your balance.

But on the flip side, when you spend your energy all the time, racking up charges and not paying it back with good quality rest, that's how you fuck up your credit. And when our energy is on bad-credit status, it makes it harder to do anything. Now you are more likely to take out them high-interest loans—leaning on caffeine and fake-ass energy drinks just to get by. But the more you lean on them energy loans, the deeper the hole you end up in—until you end up bankrupt, laid up sick, and forced to get on an energy repayment plan anyway, costing you time, money, and quality of life.

Improving Sleep Quality

There are lots of options for getting better quality sleep. The main thing is having a good conscience and being at peace in your mind. If your conscience is bothering you, it will be hard to rest. If you are overwhelmed with work, or things are stressful with your spouse, or you have an unresolved issue that keeps your mind hostage, it can (and will) definitely challenge and affect your ability to fall asleep and rest well. So, do your best to put things in order in your life, so when your head hits the pillow, you aren't kept awake by it all. Other simple sleep aids I rock with are:

- Chamomile/valerian tea is one of my go-to natural knock-out potions
- Lavender is scientifically shown to induce a relaxing effect in most people. It's one of the most common scents used in spas to create that calming aromatherapeutic environment. Just a few drops of lavender essential oil on my pillow does the trick for

me. My brain responds like one of Pavlov's dogs, going to sleep when I smell the scent of lavender.

- Alarm clocks and apps that wake you up with gentle music like Sunrise, Alarmy, and others.
- Twenty-to-thirty-minute power naps throughout the day are helpful, especially if I've got a lot going on or I didn't get a full night's sleep.
- Sleep-focused guided meditations and audiobooks work well as kind of bedtime stories for adults
- Don't sleep on those sleep masks. When you want to shut out everything and close down shop and knock all the way out, a silk sleep mask will make you feel like you got an invisible cloak on.

Energy is the money of life, and it's got to be invested and managed right to take care of you for the long haul. One of my favorite ways to unwind and slip into sleep mode is listening to rain. That's my shit. The sound of rain is so peaceful to me. I always feel like it's a special occasion when it's raining. They say it never rains in Southern California, but it be hella rainy nights in Georgia. Those thousands of little sprinkling sounds from all the raindrops and splashes on the window are hypnotic for me. Water energy is powerful like that. Whether it's being at a beach or the relaxing feeling of rain, or like when you are taking a hot shower, it's a vibe. It rains a lot in the A, but it obviously don't rain every day, so I became a digital rain collector and started creating playlists on my phone with all kinds of rain sounds. Now, by listening to recorded rain, I can make it rain every night if I want to. I collect rain sounds like a DJ collects vintage vinyl. I got hours of everything from city showers to forest rainstorms, delicate droplets to light drizzles to downpours. It's like liquid drums playing. I just pull up my rain crate playlist on my phone, hit shuffle, and it's like I'm Djing myself to sleep with a symphony of raindrops. It's so crazy how water is so strong and healing that just the sound of it has a calming and relaxing effect. And it makes sense being that I'm a water sign, a Pisces, so water is my element. Rain is so relaxing, it's become my go-to ambiance "music" when I'm up and working, too. Even while writing a lot of this book, I'd have rain rocking in my earbuds, helping me tap into my flow. Water has so much to teach as a metaphor when we're striving to be more balanced and graduate from the grip of the grind and relax into flowing with more grace and more ease. Investing in things that help you rest better is an investment in the kind of energy you're able to bring to your life—the right vibes in your room, the perfect mattress, the most fitting pillow with just the right amount of firmness and softness—having your particular comforts in place so you can relax and enjoy some quality shut-eye are all things that matter.

Hustle & Flow: Resting Between Rounds

Respecting rest isn't just about when we are sleeping. It's especially important to respect rest during our grind as well. Again, take boxing as an example. Boxing is one of the toughest sports in the world. Like Sugar Ray Leonard put it, *"You don't play boxing.... You play golf, you play tennis, but you don't play boxing." Boxing is a combat sport*. You go hard. You get in that ring with bad intentions to bring the pain and slug it out with all you got. But the thing is, when the end of the round comes and that bell rings, what happens? *You rest between rounds*. You go to your corner, get off your feet, sit down and take a breather, catch your wind, cool your head, have some water, reset, let the cut man nurse your wounds, and you listen to your corner so you can make adjustments to win the next round. That's how I, as an admitted workaholic, have learned to see taking breaks. It's the rest between rounds. You might have been standing toe-to-toe with life and handling yours or you might be on the ropes taking an ass whipping, but just before the towel gets thrown in, the bell rings. That's what taking breaks does; breaks help you stay in the fight. The quality of your rest determines the quality of your fight.

A really useful technique for bringing more flow to my workdays is the Pomodoro technique. I call it PT for short. It's a simple way to manage time when you're working on something for long hours, by breaking the workload up into bite-size chunks. In my case, I use it for things like writing books or writing and producing songs, but it can work for any and all kinds of tasks and activities that take a lot of time to finish. We workaholics tend to think that when we've got a long road of work ahead of us that the best way to get it done is to just mash the gas to the floor nonstop. No breaks. No pauses. Just go, go, go. But with the existing research, and from my own experience, I can say fasho that that's not as productive as you might believe. I used to be proud to say I put in fourteen or eighteen hours or more straight in the studio and didn't even stop once to go use the bathroom. I prided myself on having insane focus. I thought that's what it meant to have a great work ethic. But what I was really doing was working harder, not smarter. Taking breaks throughout the day actually helps you be more productive in the long run.

What's that you're thinking, my fellow hustler? How can you be more productive even though you are working less? PT is based on really dialing in and being laser focused for a preset chunk of time (like twenty-five minutes) and then giving yourself a five-minute break. That's one round. After about four rounds, which is about two hours, you take a longer break, for about fifteen to twenty minutes or so.

It works for two reasons: One is the urgency it brings to your focus. With only twenty-five minutes, you ain't dilly dallying around like you got all day to get shit done. You ain't got no time to be distracted. You have to make those 1,500 seconds count. And two, forcing yourself to retreat to the corner when the bell rings and take a five-minute rest between rounds helps cut down on that burnt-out feeling as the workday rolls on.

When that timer goes off at the end of each Pomodoro round, it snaps you out of your grind mode so you can get up and stretch or drink some water or go to the bathroom or just step away for a sec like a human being, instead of pressing on nonstop like a machine.

To do it, you can use the regular timer on your phone, but I downloaded a Pomodoro timer app 'cause it lets you easily set the timer for both the focus rounds and the rests in between. Focus Keeper is a good one if you got an iPhone, but there are a lot of them out there to choose from.

When you used to just banging out for hours straight without rest, you're probably gonna be tempted to ignore the timer and keep grinding, especially when you feel like you in a zone and you don't wanna break your stride. And shit, it's up to you to make that call. But if you really want to test it out to see how it work, you have to honor that bell when it rings and let the break work its magic. To paraphrase how Miles Davis put it, sometimes it's not the notes you play, it's the notes you don't play.

I ain't gonna front—sometimes I still keep working when the timer goes off 'cause I done already told you, I'm a grind-aholic in recovery. I've gotten a lot better, but I still wrestle with those push-it-to-the-max tendencies. But I do my best and I don't beat myself up too much about it if I'm really flowing and I just really don't want to stop. It be like that sometimes and that's alright—*sometimes*. It's about practice not perfection. And also, PT don't work in all situations like anything else. If you're in a meeting or you have appointments or you're working with other people or on other folks' schedules, you don't always have the flexibility to cut up time and breaks like that. But if you are in control of your time, it's a good tool to have; and like me when I use the Pomodoro technique, you'll be surprised how much you still can get done and how you'll feel less burnt out at the end of the day.

———

This principle of respecting rest is basically about getting better at energy management, and like any other skill, energy management is something that can be learned and improved upon. Prioritizing more sleep and taking breaks throughout the day is definitely helpful, but sometimes when you have big plans, you need even bigger energy to carry you through. And that's why the thousands-of-years-old science we about to dive into next is gonna be so dope. Check it.

CHAPTER 13

The Chi Code

"Sleep is the master of all qigong techniques." That gem right there is just one of the many powerful quotes I scribbled down in my notebook when I took a fourteen weeklong training course to learn ra qigong some years back. The course was taught by the Ausar Auset Society, an African-centered spiritual organization founded way back in 1973 by Ra Un Nefer Amen. They are based out of Brooklyn, New York, and they have over forty chapters in the US and around the world. The class was held in the historic West End neighborhood of Atlanta, upstairs in the back of a large two-story redbrick building with a couple of commercial storefronts at the front of the building. Our main instructor was a bearded Black man, a longtime member of Ausar Auset, probably somewhere in his upper forties, but you know Black don't crack. He was rocking a dope purple-and-white tie-dye dashiki and jeans. He had a simple presentation set up: a small portable table for a podium, a laptop and projector, and a PowerPoint slideshow.

Up to this point, I had only dabbled here and there with qigong. I studied *the eight pieces of brocade*, a sequence of qigong forms that looks like tai chi, that the legendary Shaolin monks practice. Nothing formal, just following along with DVDs and various online teachings a little bit. I'd been wanting to make the time in my schedule to take a full qigong course since I'd had that crazy experience with energy back in New York. And class was now in session. I sat my thermos of hot tea down on the floor and hit record on my phone as soon as the class started 'cause I didn't wanna miss shit. I can't even fully do justice to the value I got from the course in the scope of this book, so I'mma try to give you the key takeaways, but trust, it was two words: game changing.

Ra: African Roots of Qigong

There are hundreds of different schools and styles of qigong, from the qigong that Shaolin Warrior monks have practiced in monasteries in China for thousands of years, to the more simplified modern qigong practices that complement standard hospital procedures in Asia and even some cancer-treatment centers and hospitals in the US. And they all have their own different methods and uses and benefits. But the most standout thing about this particular approach to qigong practice, ra qigong, is the blend of traditional-Chinese-medicine theory and Taoist life science with African spiritual perspectives from ancient Egypt.

Ra qigong is a sequence of fourteen breathing exercises and postures combined with healing sounds you learn how to make that all help you improve the health of your internal organs and build up your energy and vitality in your everyday life, but it's way more than that. Right off the bat, just from the first few slides, we learned that qigong is two words: *chi* or *qi*, which means energy, and *gong*, which means to put in work at something or to practice over time to develop skill. A gong can last two weeks, one hundred days, or a lifetime. Chi is your life-force energy. Some people be like, "Do you believe in chi?" But it's nothing spooky to believe in; it's real, just like electricity or gravity. Chi is just vital energy. Whether you want to call it chi or not, it's the energetic waves that keep you, and everything else in the world, moving, functioning, and alive. It's in us and in everything around us. Chi is your inner live wire. It's like a living electric current that powers your life. Everything growing and thriving and living is the proof and the evidence that chi is real.

No chi, no life.

Different cultures call it by different names. In Japan, it's called *ki*. In China, of course it's *chi,* sometimes spelled *qi*. In India, it's called *prana*. Hawaiians call it *mana*. What blew me away was learning that this science was also practiced in Africa, in ancient Egypt, thousands of years before it was introduced to Asian cultures. Chi, in their culture, was embodied in the concept of *ra*.

Redefining Ra

Now, you might've heard that Ra was the name of the sun god that Egyptians worshipped. If you search for it now, you'll see that all over the net. But our instructor taught us that this is a false idea. He said that myth came from Eurocentric Egyptologists who didn't understand the rich complexities of African culture.

We looked at slides of hieroglyphic images that revealed to us that the sun, as in the solar disk in the sky, was actually called Aten, not Ra. Aten was the specific ancient Egyptian term for the sun in the sky, and it was Pharaoh Akhenaten who changed his name from

THE EYE OF RA

So, we know that we live in a solar system, right? That of course means our Earth and our lives literally revolve around the sun. The people of Kemet, an older term for ancient Egypt, were some of the world's first scientists, and they recognized the central role that the sun plays in sustaining life. Everything that is alive depends on the energy of the sun. Plants use sunlight to make energy and animals

Amenhotep to Akhenaten, which means something like "to elevate the sun," when he converted to sun worship, so the story goes. Our instructor explained that this is where the false notion came from that our ancestors in ancient Egypt were sun worshippers. He added that those myths have been repeated over and over by Egyptologists who don't really know the real deal Holyfield or who have agendas to hide the truth, if they do know what's up. These insights were so deep and interesting and eye-opening. I was writing all this shit down, filling up my notebook with gem after gem.

In ancient Egyptian culture, ra is *related* to the sun, *but it's not the sun. Ra symbolizes the truth, describing how the energy relationship that the sun has with all forms of life is equivalent to how the energy in our bodies works to promote our well-being.* Ra expresses the understanding that our vitality, chi, or life force is interconnected to the sun, functioning similarly in our bodies. Egyptians didn't worship the sun. They understood that we are solar systems ourselves.

I ain't gonna front, it seems like some complex shit at first, but once I took the time to study and absorb and process it, it's simpler than it seems, and it's worth nerding out a li'l bit to catch the jewels.

eat plants, or eat other animals who eat plants, and convert that stored sunlight into energy. Then we eat those plants or animals and convert that stored sunlight into energy. We depend on the sun. But not just for energy. We are deeply connected to the sun's rhythm and way of being.

As the sun rises and sets every day, we are deeply affected. It regulates us so much that we have our own inner solar clock, called the circadian rhythm. The term *cir-cadian* comes from the Latin words *circa*, meaning "about," and *dies*, which means "day." Circadian rhythms exist in all types of organisms. They help flowers open and close at the right time and keep bears from coming out of hibernation too soon. They keep nocturnal animals from leaving their shelter during the day when doing so would expose them to more predators. In humans, circadian rhythms coordinate our mental and physical systems throughout our bodies like hormone release and regulation, energy production, growth, digestion, elimination, repairs, and literally everything else under the sun—pardon the pun. The many different circadian rhythms throughout the body are all connected to a "master clock" in the hypothalamus—the part of your brain that controls your autonomic nervous system—which sends signals at different times of the day (and night) to regulate activity throughout the body.

By nature's supreme design, the eyes play a key role in the process. Both the eyes and the hypothalamus are highly sensitive to light, so sunlight serves as an external cue and regulator that enters through our eyes and influences the signals (hormones and chemicals) that the hypothalamus sends to coordinate all the other internal clocks in the body. For this reason, circadian rhythms are closely connected to the cycle of light and dark, day and night. There are certain inner processes that only happen in the daytime when you are up and awake and active, and then there are certain internal functions that only happen overnight when you're asleep, like we learned in the last chapter. Exercise or the light on your phone screen or even temperature can affect the master clock, but sunlight is the most powerful influence on circadian rhythms.

Now look at how genius our ancestors were in encoding this knowledge in the hieroglyph for ra. One of the most-used hieroglyphs for ra is an eye! The hypothalamus is that "eye" of ra in man. Since we this deep in the rabbit hole now, you might as well chew on this linguistic nugget while we here: the Spanish word for the sun is *sol*. Kinda makes you say "Hmmm" when you consider all of this in the context of the phrase *The eyes are the window to the soul*. And not to mention how similar the sound and energetic meaning of the words *solar, cellular,* and *soul* are. They each speak to sources of life force energy and activity.

Shit is deep, yo. Some studies show when people are sunlight deprived, they experience symptoms of depression. Seasonal affective disorder (SAD) is a type of depression related to changes in seasons. For most people who suffer from SAD, it usually begins in the fall and continues into the winter months (when there is less light), and the effects are a sapping away of energy, dark gloomy feelings, and moodiness. Sunlight prompts the brain to produce serotonin, a hormone that wakes us up, gives us energy, and makes us feel good. That same serotonin gets converted into melatonin at night, and that's the chemical concoction that makes you feel that sleepy sensation before you doze off. Our energy and life force are solar powered. If we want to have lots of energy every day and continue to grow and thrive, it's only natural for us to sync our activities, cycles, rhythms, and habits with the sun's cycles and seasons. It's not sun worship; the sun is a part of us.

Wu Ji

My "chi IQ" was literally rising like the sun as I worked on the exercises during the fourteen-week course. We learned specific dietary tips similar to intermittent fasting to maximize daily energy production and various beneficial effects of a regular qigong practice for improving the function of the immune system, digestion, blood flow, and other vital systems of the body.

We learned about the Five Elements Theory of energy regeneration called the Wuxing and how it works in the organs, emotions, and in life, and we explored some of the deep metaphoric and philosophical wisdom it contains. Each element is symbolic of a phase of the cyclical energy-generation process. Water feeds wood, wood feeds fire, fire creates earth, earth creates metal, metal's condensation creates water, and the cycle repeats. These phases correspond to how energy works universally. It was a crash course in energy management that was everything I had hoped it would be and so much more.

Each week after the lecture portion of our class, for the rest of our three-hour sessions, we'd remove our shoes, move our chairs to the rear of the room to make space for everyone to spread out arm's-length apart, and get in some group practice with the instructor's guidance through the fourteen postures and breathing exercises.

There are a lot of little details to the practice and so much to remember, so I had come up with a strategy for memorizing and practicing at home to get a better hold on the elements of the system and try to simplify my learning curve.

I sat down at my desk and first identified the three main parts of the practice: the postures, the procedures, and the healing sounds you make while doing them. Then I started creating a study plan with index cards. I wrote the name of a posture on the front of an index card, and then on the back I put the phonetic spelling of the sound to train myself to memorize which healing sound goes with each posture. Afya helped quiz me until I could remember them all.

I would often practice the forms outside in our backyard in the early morning—barefoot on the grass while facing sunward, surrounded by our wooden deck and our raised garden bed, looking over a natural fence of rosemary bushes, clumping bamboo shrubs, and an eighty-pound stone buddha statue. I had researched and downloaded a timer app that not only had all the functions that allowed me to program the names and timing of the movements, but it even spoke the names out load. This meant I didn't have to break form or concentration to check my phone for which posture came next.

All fourteen of the postures are anchored in a basic stance called wu ji. This super simple stance has so much power and depth of meaning. You're basically standing up, facing forward, with just a slight bend in your knees. Not deep like a squat, but just enough to create a little bit of tension in your legs. Not too much. Then, you sit your hips back as if there is a tall stool behind you that is holding you up. Keep your arms relaxed by your side with about a tennis ball's worth of space under your armpits. And just hold all that, breathing in and out through the nose, staying relaxed with that little bit of tension in your legs. That's wu ji. It's like a form of standing meditation in and of itself. You can hold it for a few minutes as a warm-up or you can hold it for a full hour or more if you dare, as a full workout.

The term *wu li* means void, nothingness, neutral, limitless, without polarity. It means avoiding extremes. Neutral. Natural. It's the first step in the journey of a thousand miles on the path of qigong, and it embodies the jewel of balance. The most important aspect of wu li standing posture is to relax. Yeah, you're using effort to stand, so there's a slight tension that you are maintaining, but the point is to stand strong while at the same time staying relaxed. That's also a great takeaway for life, learning how to stand strong and handle your business but also how to balance strength and form with relaxation. Respect rest. Balance is key.

Chi Is Everything

As I worked and memorized my forms over the days and weeks to come, I could feel changes in my energy levels and I was getting more sensitive to my intuition. I started pairing and alternating my usual morning meditation and neighborhood runs with "chi-up" sessions, and I noticed I was steadier in my pacing on my jogs. I was having more insightful downloads, and creative ideas were flowing like water. Things just seemed "easier." It's hard to explain, but I was feeling "lighter," less tension in my body and mind, and it seemed like serendipitous things were occurring that started to make me wonder if I was actually tapping into the Star Wars force after all. Shit, who knows—maybe George Lucas was studying traditional Chinese energy theories when he wrote Star Wars! Either way, I was lit! I might don't have no lightsaber but learning how to manage my energy better became a lifesaver.

As I studied my notes and did more research and practiced in my regular everyday life, I came to another huge aha moment:

Everything Is Qigong.

Those same five qualities of the Wuxing—water, wood, fire, earth, and metal—correspond to the characteristics of the seasons: winter, spring, summer, late summer, and autumn. One of the most significant seasonal-alignment practices that I picked up from the Ausar Auset teachings was doing a certain set of rituals around the winter solstice every year with my family. Winter corresponds with the water principle, so it's a time to return to balance and rest and water our life force with extra sleep, fasting, meditation, and visualization. This is the time we make our vision boards for the year to come. This is when we digitally detox and focus on high vibrational reading and spiritual- and personal-growth content. The first year we all watched *The Secret*, did yin yoga, and made vision boards at the dining-room table. It was beautiful. The ritual brings us all together as a family and recharges us for the year to come with renewed energy to spring forth into the new year. Timing this relaxation period with the winter season is as powerful and as natural as planting seeds in their appropriate planting season. It's the perfect opportunity to take advantage of the natural forces that are present and moving in harmony with that solar clock that makes us thrive.

Chi is life force; it's the mechanism of everything unfolding in our lives. The five phases are the very blueprint that all-natural processes and phenomena in the known universe follow. Knowing how energy functions allows you to learn how to harness it and make use of it in more skillful ways. Life energy, my energy, your energy don't just function randomly; there's a specific sequence of generation and regeneration. Qigong has helped me start to look at things happening in my body and life with a higher chi IQ. With this framework I am better able to recognize, read, and ride the energetic flux and signature stages that show up in all kinds of situations and circumstances in my life.

Learning about the nuts and bolts of how the energy of life operates is a gold mine for personal well-being, and the Wuxing model is an energy cheat sheet, a master key that unlocks how physical and emotional health and vitality are maintained.

Managing Your Chi to Manage Your Stress

The hustle and bustle of modern life is stressful, and that stress can be difficult to live with. Many people experience chronic stress anxiety.

Symptoms like insomnia and depression are far too common. Besides the mental pressure, there's also a physical toll. Research has linked stress with a variety of unhealthy conditions, including heart disease, obesity, and diabetes. Western medicine tends to look at stress symptoms separately with measures to treat symptoms one by one. Traditional Chinese medicine (TCM) takes a more holistic approach, focusing on root causes instead of just branch symptoms.

TCM considers the state and strength of the patient's chi, that vital life force or energy that flows through every living thing. When your chi is strong and balanced, it flows freely throughout your body. It carries energy to every cell, and it helps all your organs and tissues communicate effectively with each other.

When chi is low, we feel drained and exhausted, our hormones get out of whack, and we get sick easier. If left unresolved for long periods of time, small issues can become massive problems and chronic diseases affecting the heart, liver, kidneys, and digestive system. The main cause of chi deficiency is usually one or more of the following: lack of sleep, dehydration, poor diet, lack of loving relationships, poor air quality, stress, substance abuse, allergic reactions, and not enough of the right kind of exercise.

Therapies and practices like qigong, acupuncture, and reiki are designed to restore chi, which leads to actual healing of root issues and results in greater health for the whole body. The good news is that you can raise your chi with simple natural practices like eating in a healthful way, exercising and relaxing regularly, breathing intentionally and deeply, keeping your stress low, meditating, and staying optimistic and joyful about your life. After all, in many cases, chi becomes unbalanced, blocked, and deficient as a result of unskillful management of emotions and high levels of stress. The practice of meditation has been thoroughly researched and there are tons of evidence-based studies demonstrating its benefits.

———

Since I have included meditation as part of my regular routine, I'm better able to manage negative emotions when they come up. Instead of always feeling too exhausted and overwhelmed to manage life's challenges, I use restorative tools that help me recharge my energy and sustain my endurance to flow better. I have better whole-body health, a stronger immune system, easier healing after injuries, and increased mental calm. I use qigong strategies as one of many methods of stress relief, as an exercise modality to use when I take breaks in my workday, to assist my body in healing, to shift my state of mind, to bring more energy to my runs, and to keep up with my youngest son who has energy in spades! I'm always returning to the five-phases framework for exploring how I feel and what is going on around me. For instance, if I'm irritable, I'll equate that energetically with fire and I know that water puts out fire, so I will go take a shower or listen to rain sounds or take a walk along the creek near my house, or even just drink a glass of water or hot tea. Likening emotions to natural forces of nature and responding accordingly helps me reconnect with my flow and peace. If I'm kind of scatterbrained and I need to gather my thoughts and focus and concentrate, I will equate that to needing to be in a more grounded (earth like) and concentrated (metal like) state of mind.

One solution is to sit down and create specific categories, gathering my ideas into a journal, note or document and organize each thought within distinct parameters, giving structure to the chaos. I create schedules to hold myself accountable by using the metal like concentrating principle for focusing.

Even the framework of this book is aligned with the sustainable energy model I learned from qigong. The Wuxing reveals the master pattern of how all things flow, change, happen, and unfold in the world. The five-phases system underlies everything: celestial patterns, historical events, social structures, businesses and economies, personal relationships, political strategies, moral philosophies, personality expressions, daily energy fluctuations, medical treatments and everything else imaginable that moves and changes. The science of qigong is a deep well of wisdom that can only be mastered from a lifelong journey of practice, but you don't have to master qigong to start being more skillful with using and replenishing your energy. If you respect and go with the way of energy, you will generate power and energy in your life because the checks and balances of the cycle make it so that it replenishes itself sustainably and naturally. Look at how many billions of years the earth has been following the same patterns to sustain life. If we go against the way of energy and don't respect the checks and balances, we will deplete and drain ourselves and lack the power and energy to thrive in our lives.

Trust me, that alopecia patch I had is not a good look. Respecting rest, getting better quality sleep, and learning how energy works has been fruitful in my life garden. See what might sprout up from it in yours. Start to recognize what drains your energy and minimize and/or avoid those people, places, thoughts, and things. Don't hustle yourself to death. Trust in the abundance. The universe got you, homey. It's health over hustle. Even the sun respects stillness—that's what the solstice is. Stillness recharges our batteries and regenerates our energy. Keeping your wheel of life in balance is what creates the optimum conditions for your energy to flow and flourish in your life.

CHAPTER 14

R&R (Relaxation and Recreation)

Nurturing myself is not selfish, it's essential to my
survival and well-being and those I love.
—*"Manifestival" mantra*

Each of the red dirt–road communities that made up my original stomping grounds in the rural town of Shadeville—Wakulla
County—Florida, were mostly dense woodlands populated by small
pockets of related families living on shared plots of land. A few years
back, my pops gifted me research documents he compiled on his
side of the family that show we have lived in those same necks of the
woods since the 1800s. My great grandfather Papa Luke Smith was a
local hero in Wakulla. He looked like an older version of Dapper Dan
minus the Harlem flamboyance, bald on top with some white scruff
on the sides and thin wire-frame glasses. He worked as a boatman
at Wakulla Springs, a local natural resort, taking tours of folks out
on glass-bottom boat exhibitions to explore the local marine wildlife
and habitat. The highlight of a day at the Springs was Papa Luke's
tour, where he would take you out on the river and turn off the engine
and everything would get real quiet. Papa Luke would start to whis-
tle and sing his song, "Ol' Henry," which was the nickname he had
for a colorful local species of fish that appeared when he'd sing (and

perhaps discreetly sprinkle some food over the side of the boat) as if they responded to his call. People loved him for this, 'cause it made the ride special.

Those glass-bottom boat rides at Wakulla Springs were magical times. Every time he'd sing that song, sure enough the Ol' Henry would show up. He made you feel that you too were connected with nature. Growing up, I had a lot of men around me that inspired and encouraged my love for the outdoors. One of my most treasured memories is time spent with my uncle Bo, who introduced me to archery in the backwoods of those same Wakulla roads. Uncle Bo isn't actually my uncle—we are actually third or fourth cousins—but he was like an uncle to me. He used to take me with him on hunting adventures. He used to pick me up from my aunt's house over "in the hole," as our family neighborhood was affectionately called, and we'd walk miles up the soft sand-dirt road toward the "rock bottom" section of our community into the forest areas behind his mobile trailer home. Uncle Bo and I would use bows and arrows and pellet guns to go hunting for squirrels and birds. I remember feeling too tall and too close to the low ceiling inside Uncle Bo's small single-wide trailer kitchen, but it didn't matter because I always had the time of my life hanging out with him. Uncle Bo was a marksman with the bow and the gun, and I picked up tips from him while I tagged along.

We'd spend hours out on the hunt. Every now and then we'd lodge an arrow or pellet in our prey and listen for the thump they'd make when they fell out of the tree and onto the forest floor. We'd gather our kill of birds and squirrels—mostly squirrels—and take them back to the trailer to cook up. For every squirrel you shot, you got to cut the tail off and clip it to the back of your hat. I remember one time I had a red-and-white trucker cap with the bib cocked up with like four bushy gray tails clipped to the back. Yes sir, we was country AF!

Uncle Bo let me help him skin and clean our catch. If you are vegan and you are triggered by hunting details, you might want to skip this part. I remember how light their bodies felt, about the same weight as a bottle of water. In a biology-field-trip kind of way, it was disturbing but interesting for me to participate in the process. The lifeless squirrels we hunted would go from having fuzzy, whiskery, grayish-brown backsides and velvety white bellies to being boiled and de-furred to reveal the little slick salmon-pink meat suits underneath. Then those limp pink bodies would be beheaded, gutted, and rinsed thoroughly under the cold tap water in the sink until they were blood free. Then they'd be chopped into the choice parts, flour-dusted white, dropped into the hot crackling Crisco grease, and fried up golden brown.

Uncle Bo would smother his fried squirrel with hot sauce, so I would follow suit—and, yes, if you're wondering, it tasted just like chicken. It may seem gruesome today to some but hunting for food with the bow is one of the oldest human activities there is.

Going on these kinds of archery adventures as a kid meant everything to me. It wasn't until I was in my late thirties that archery came back into my life. My oldest son, Afya, and I were visiting at our Rasta homegirl Moon's crib for her daughter Zenijah's birthday party, and I met and got to chopping it up with this bro Jhavaun Green. We hit it off immediately, and I found he was a man of many pursuits and skills, one of them being he was an archery coach and founder of the National Black Archers Association. He gave me his self-published book on archery and explained he initially got into archery because his daughter wanted to try it. Being the awesome father that he is, the next thing he knew he was engulfed in it himself and had become an instructor. He felt compelled to make the sport more accessible to people of color. As we chatted, I felt that old-school nostalgia of what archery had meant to me as a youth resurfacing. His passion for using archery to connect with his daughter reminded me of my connection with my uncle Bo. So, I decided to take him up on his offer for a free lesson.

I drove up to Lithonia, just a ways outside of east Atlanta, to meet

Jhavaun for my lesson. When I got out my ride, I saw him all Afro, beard, and smiles next to a section of orange cones he had set up in the open field, marking off what would be our range lanes. There were a few rows of circular archery targets with the yellow, blue, and red bull's-eyes printed on them set up on either side of the cones about thirty feet south of us. Over the duration of the session, I got a wonderful tutorial on the basics of handling a bow and arrow safely and got reacquainted with the fundamental mechanics of shooting. Before I knew it, the time had gone by and I'd even landed some great groups of shots along the way. But what I noticed more than anything was I hadn't cared too much about how many bull's-eyes I'd hit; I just enjoyed being there, meditatively practicing the techniques he instructed me on, feeling the breeze and the sun, and fellowshipping with the homey. I remember thinking to myself, *Oh, this is what people mean when they say they got a fun hobby. I think I found me one.*

That first lesson felt so natural to me and so fun and relaxing that I instantly felt like I needed to do it more as a way to unwind and give me other things to do besides grind all the time. So, I continued training over the next weeks and months when I could make the time, and after a while Jhavaun suggested I consider taking the instructor course. I didn't want to become an instructor to take on any clients per se (Where's the time?) but I thought it might be a great way to support his organization, which I felt was a great cause. It would also be a great way for me to gain more practice and detailed knowledge about the sport, so I agreed to take the course. After weeks of practice and some technical book study, I took my test in Lithonia with about five other students from around the country. Not to bore you with bragging, but ya boy ended up with the highest scores of our testing group. I completed both the USA Archery Level 1 and Level 2 instructor courses in the same day, and I've been enjoying archery again as an adult in my leisure time ever since.

ARCHERY GOES WAY BACK

The bow and the arrow have been a part of our survival as a species since day one of their invention. Archery has been continuously practiced on the African continent throughout all of human history. *Ta-Seti*, which means "land of the bow," was the name given to the area of Nubia in Africa by the ancient Egyptians because Nubians were so skilled in archery. Nubia's most traded and valuable commodities, like ivory and animal hides, came from their bow-hunting skills. The Egyptians wrote that the Nubians were the best of the best with the bow and arrow and recruited them into their armies.

Archaeologists discovered a beautifully painted, well-preserved wooden model of Nubian archers in an ancient Egyptian tomb. The forty-man, lean and mean squadron of Afro-rocking, brown-skinned figures are marching in stride, each holding a bow in one hand and a bunch of arrows in the other. I wonder how exciting that was for the archaeologists to discover such a beautiful wooden carving of Black archers. I would've had to put that shit in my house, sorry.

Farther south in the motherland, researchers uncovered well-preserved arrowheads in South African caves that are more than 64,000 years old. The Ethiopian Maya, the Botswana Bushmen of the Kalahari, and the Maasai tribe of Kenya are still living practitioners of the unsung African heritage of archery. In almost every culture—all over the Americas, the Caribbean, Europe, Australia, Asia, and beyond—somewhere down the line, everyone has a connection to archery in their lineage. Since it requires intricate planning, material collection, tool preparation, a range of knowledge of the environment, good timing instincts, as well as applied physics, archery not only provided food, clothing, and defense, it also became a teaching tool. I imagine from my own experiences with archery that all the while it also provided our ancestors a relaxing form of recreation and fellowship, too.

Letting the Arrow Go

Archery is a great metaphor for the need for balance between tension and relaxation. The bow is a firm stick that wants to be straight, but it is bent and held under a lot of tension by the bowstring. When you notch your arrow and pull it back with the bowstring, that tension is transferred and multiplied into the string with pounds and pounds of pressure that is locked, loaded, and ready to be released, launching that arrow like a rocket through space into the target. One of the standout insights I came to learn over time might sound strange, but it's totally true: you always hit what you aim at. Every single time, without fail, in archery you always hit exactly what you're aiming for. It's impossible to miss. The key is to know the difference between what you think you are aiming at and what you're actually aiming at, because the results don't lie. That arrow goes exactly where it's sent. That's your true aim. What we call misses are not errors of our arrows missing our target, it's lack of clarity of our aim.

Archery teaches you about your true aim. And life is the same way. We get the results we get every time because we're not actually aiming at what we think we're aiming for, but the results don't lie. Being of true aim means clarifying your intention so you can truly have your best shot at life.

An archery bow can hold anywhere from twenty to upwards of

seventy pounds or more of pressure. That release takes all that pressure and focuses it and unleashes it into the arrow that travels at dazzling speeds, wobbling and arching and piercing deep into the target of your true aim.

When it comes to archery as a means of rest and relaxation, that's the true aim. It's not about obsessing over bull's-eyes. It's not about keeping score. It's about having fun, forgetting about work, forgetting about the past, the future, issues, and problems, and just being a kid again at play.

Archery gets its name from how the arrows travel in an arching pattern to the target. The skill is about making considerations in your posture and aim that take into account the way the tension of the bow and string plays into the powerful freedom of the arrow to follow its natural course.

That's what hobbies are all about, and that's why they are so necessary. Our daily grind is like that stiff bow that bends us out of shape. Pulling the bowstring is like the effort it takes to stretch ourselves out of a tightly wound work mode and get in position to fully let go. Doing our hobbies, whatever they may be, is that release of the string that lets us free up, fly free for a bit, and hit our target of joy, relaxation, and play.

There's a point when you have to ask yourself: Are you living to work or working to live? Stress can show up in a lot of ways. It can drain your energy, shorten your temper, weaken your immune system, depress your mind, and negatively influence your decisions. When life gets too overwhelming, having hobbies can minimize stress, reinspire and reinvigorate you, and help you relax. Doing things we really enjoy outside of work supports mental fitness and lowers anxiety, stress, and irritability. Hobbies give us an escape from the grind. Some of my most relaxing hobbies and activities these days are archery, jogging, steam rooms, forest walks, long hot showers, and reading.

Keeping Yourself in Balance

> You ain't got to catch a flight to catch a vibe
> A getaway don't have to be far away homey, we outside
> —*Stic "Lace Up"*

What I've learned for sure from Afya's coaching on the wheel of life is that I enjoy life more when I'm more mindful of balance and not too overwhelmed by extremes. I've made a lot of progress in being more mindful about recognizing when I'm getting out of balance, and I know how to take steps to return myself to balance sooner, but it's still a challenge because my grind ethic is so ingrained in how I roll.

Case in point is a recent time I was feeling out of balance. It had been one of the heaviest, emotionally intense years of my life, and as stress kept compounding, I knew deep down I needed to take some time to get away—just for a few days. A getaway would help me recalibrate and recharge and come back revitalized, I reasoned. But as awesome as that sounds, it wasn't an easy decision. I've traveled around the world, taken Afya and our sons on many excursions internationally and domestically, but in over twenty years, I had never taken any solo vacays. Like ever. Afya gave me her blessing, but even though I knew I needed it, part of me still felt guilty leaving her to handle the everyday load of parenting a rambunctious toddler and caring for all the household duties and business that made up our blessed but busy lives at the time. It felt weird to try to relax somewhere, knowing the weight it would add to Afya's shoulders when I was away. Of course, I've traveled a lot for work as a world-touring hip-hop artist but that comes with my role as a provider, so I'm okay with being away for business. But traveling solo for leisure—I'm still working on being okay with that. I just never allowed or afforded that kind of time for myself.

We'd be on tour and the guys would often stay a few days after the gig to hang out in the city we'd stopped in to take in more of the local sights and have fun before they got back to their families, but not me. And I mean not EVER. In fact, my de facto MO would be for our tour manager to book me on the first thing smokin' in the morning. Even if I was getting offstage at 2:00 a.m., I'd almost always have a 6:00 a.m. flight to get back home and share the load as soon as physically possible. Fans would see me vanish as soon as we finished "Hip Hop." I would sometimes take a few pictures or sign a few autographs but I wasn't interested in hanging around too much. I'd give my all to the performance and before the crowd was finished cheering, I'd be in the green room ready to move, collect my things in the hotel, and be at the airport first thing. So, planning a solo getaway was not an easy thing for me, but I decided that if I was going to strive for more balance in my life, there was no time like the present to make it happen.

———

Since it was fall and getting colder every day in the A, I wanted to go somewhere hot. I was trying to decide between a familiar fun spot like Miami and somewhere that I'd never been. I planned on only being gone three or four days so that ruled out any international destinations. I thought about Austin, Texas, because I've had some great experiences there. As I kept searching, I remembered I'd heard that when Louis Farrakhan was deathly ill some years back, he went to Arizona to heal up because of the high quality of the desert air. Something in me resonated with the thought of being in the desert, and I knew just who to call.

I gave my boy Pree, an actor, fitness coach, and entrepreneur who lives in Phoenix, a ring to check the vibes and ask him about the local haps. I'd met Pree at a six-week series of outdoor wellness events I hosted in the A, called the Outsiders. Both Pree and I, being the passionate workaholics and visionaries that we are, took the idea of a simple weekend getaway of relaxation to the next level. That call became the seed to something much larger. Before we got off the phone, we had planned a weeklong men's wellness retreat—I called it the "Manifestival"—with fourteen of my homies from around the country. All of the guys are brothers who are good friends of mine, some I've known for decades, and are movers and shakers in their own right. Our Manifestival crew consisted of a medley of fathers, filmmakers, photographers, life coaches, touring managers, restaurant owners, actors, producers, real-estate investors, football players, clothing designers, finance advisors, tech developers, educators, fashion designers, shamans, entrepreneurs, hip-hop artists, and creatives. I invited each of the guys personally because I thought we'd all gel well together and become a powerful networking tribe. I just knew that each individual personality would make the experience uplifting and enjoyable.

We rented a nine-room mansion with an infinity pool in the valley of the Sedona desert and set an agenda, including hiking, archery, running, martial arts, mountain climbing, and canyon strolls, and time to kick back and go with the flow. It was our unique version of a guy's getaway to kick it and have fun and enjoy the break from our everyday grizzles.

As the days rolled closer to the event, the guys started individually hitting me to gauge the vibes on documenting different aspects of the trip. The filmmakers and photographers of the crew were especially interested in creating content from our outing, but a grind-aholic recognizes a grind-aholic, and I was determined that if the trip was actually gonna work as intended, I knew we couldn't turn the trip into anything that would end up being too much like "work." All these bros taking a retreat to invest in our self-care is a rarity, and I understood and shared the excitement and the validity of capturing some footage, but I wanted to make sure that we were all going to prioritize being present and actually getting rest and not become too engrossed in creating content out of our experiences. So, we made a compromise that filming and photography would be fine so long as it doesn't interfere with the number-one code of the trip: Respect rest!

Pree volunteered to host us and facilitate the logistics for our small army of bredren. I put together our trip itinerary with beautiful photos of our luxurious accommodations and set the tone with the headline:

NOURISHING YOURSELF IS NOT SELFISH;
IT'S ESSENTIAL TO YOUR SURVIVAL AND
WELL-BEING AND THOSE YOU LOVE.

It was a full trip. I got my partners at Diadora to bless the whole squad with fresh sneakers and jackets, pants, and socks, and I gifted all the guys with hardcover copies of Will Smith's memoir. Pree gifted us all a book on how manifesting works. We ate Ethiopian food and Jamaican food, drank green juices, and snacked on fruit while connecting and getting acquainted. These were all friends of mine but many of them were meeting each other for the first time. It was great to see the natural brotherly chemistry happening amongst the homies.

We climbed Camelback Mountain—which was challenging but invigorating—settling at about halfway up because it was getting dark and we didn't want to make our way back down in the dark. The mountain safety team kept emphasizing how dangerous it would be to try to come down in the dark. I even caught my good friend Radhz, stopping him from falling, when he slipped on our way down, so it was good we listened. Back at the bottom, we sealed the deal with some group calisthenics—one hundred push-ups done in clips of ten with ten-second rests in between—all in unison. This gave us all a nice pump and a feeling of collective victory.

We enjoyed four days of comradery, uplifting convos, relaxation, and fun. The homey Jhavaun led our archery activities with our local brother Kylon who heads up the Arizona-based Vanguard Initiative—a local archery program that makes archery more accessible to youth and people of color. My boy Crisanto is a cool-ass Filipino DJ, producer, and videographer. He's also a kundalini yoga instructor, so he led the morning yoga practice. My mentor since I was kicked out of school way back, Alan Floyd, led us on some inspiring musical meditations, spiritual musings, and hilarious moments. The bro Radhz, who is also a minister and life coach @teamhayesTLP, added on brilliantly with his message about taking the limits off our visions of how awesome our lives can be when we elevate our mindsets to expect the best. Pree led us into the mountains and guided us through a powerful group meditation as we sat high up in the cliffs of Amitabha Stupa and Peace Park, chanting oms to reinforce our intentions overlooking the city. We had fireside chats by the infinity pool. We mapped the constellations with an app on one of the guys' phones. Beats got made. Chess got played. We worked the gloves and hand mitts, shot some hoops, and went on dusty dirt-road runs. I made coconut vegetable soup for the guys on one day and my homey Jermaine made spaghetti the next. Dave Dread, Von, Curtis, and everyone else added to the convos with great energy that made the Manifestival trip a success. It was absolutely wonderful.

On the final day, something happened that almost never happens in the desert—it rained all day. It was a special closing to a special convergence. We all shared our vision and top goals for the coming year and pledged our collective support to help each of us manifest these visions into being. I'm so grateful for those times together, and I can't wait to do it again. We can get so accustomed to living with the stress of the grind but I've found that we really have to prioritize and protect our joy by doing things that keep us nourished spiritually, mentally, and physically.

We have to keep stress at bay by being just as serious about play.

Making It Real: Hobbies Energize Our Health

Finding the right activities and hobbies for you is an art in itself. Hobbies will surely benefit your life, but not every hobby will be a good fit for you. Choosing a hobby is all about realizing what interests you outside of your daily grind and work life. If you work sitting down at a desk all day, hunched over on a laptop, or thumbing away on a phone but you love being physically active, maybe you would like a hobby that allows you to indulge more in your active side. On the other hand, if your job involves a lot of physical activity or manual labor, then you might want more relaxing hobbies that channel your Zen mode, since doing less activity might be more suitable to you. Hobbies help you do positive things with your time—you know how they say idle hands are the devil's workshop. I wonder how many people who are always recreationally drinking and drugging are really just bored and haven't taken the time to find healthier things to do. I bet a lot.

Hobbies are flexible. They can either be done with others or as solo endeavors. You can do yoga with a class or alone, following along with a YouTube video. Cooking can be a way to unwind and be creative and relax if it's not something you already do for a living or need a break from. Volunteering offers hobby opportunities that help others. There are so many ways to step your hobby game up.

If you're struggling with choosing at least one hobby to pick up, it's worth taking the time to really consider, even write down what kinds of activities you feel most drawn to. It's never too late fam. Explore and try different shit. You might discover a new activity that really elevates the quality of your life.

With the work-life shifts created by the COVID-19 pandemic, more and more of us are working from the crib than ever, so the distinction between our work and play schedule is becoming less and less clear. Having hobbies, now more than ever, helps us maintain a clear balance between our professional pursuits and our personal lives so we're not spending every single second of the day focused on the hustle. Even if you took up meditation as a new hobby, you might discover more than you imagine.

To really integrate this into your life, do the wheel-of-life assessment once a month, or at least quarterly, so you don't go too long without recalibrating yourself. Plan some regular time for yourself to take a break from routines and indulge in some fun time with your loved ones throughout the year. Also squeeze in some solo days here and there as well, at least once a month or so.

Every now and then it's a good idea to take digital fasts and lay off social media for a few days at a time. Taking a break from tech gives us a chance to recharge our own batteries and helps us feel more mindful and aware of our surroundings. If you do need to stay on your phone or computer, use the screen dimmer on your devices and consider getting a pair of blue-light-blocking glasses—even when you're just scrolling and not working. A good rule of thumb is to fast, take some time off, and recalibrate at least once a season. Learning to practice detachment will go a long way in keeping your stress low.

Your flow could look something like this:

- Daily me time
- Biweekly pedicure
- Monthly massage
- Quarterly friends
- Annually family vacay

But as with everything, do what works best for you. Take breaks—mash the brake so you don't break. If you ever question the power of breaks, remember that's what hip-hop was founded on: highlighting the breaks. The breakbeat sections of songs are the best part. Get outside and take advantage of the moments. The rest between rounds is important, so listen to your corner.

CONSISTENCY

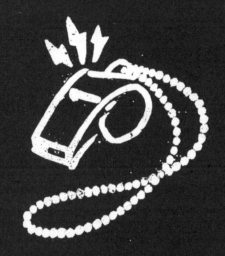

CHAPTER 15

Renaissance

Inspiration is found everywhere if you look hard
enough.

—*RZA*

S o far, we've journeyed through four elemental principles. We dipped
our feet in the water, studying the principle of knowledge and the
value of learning every day and continuing to grow and evolve. We
discussed strategies for mental fitness, while we strive to keep a white-
belt mentality as we flow with the way of life.

We've grounded ourselves like plants in the earth by listening to
our guts, gathering nutrition and hydration insights from the rainforest to nourish ourselves like a thriving ecosystem.

We chewed on the fruits of finding our own paths in fitness and
building strength, flexibility, endurance, and vitality like the wood
element, like rooted trees growing, branching out, blooming, and
blossoming. We appreciated the personal growth that fitness fertilizes
beyond the physical.

We challenged and counseled our inner beast mode to appreciate
inner peace mode. We discussed working smarter instead of harder,
respecting rest, and working mindfully with our chi to keep the grind

aligned with peace of mind so our vitality stays golden and solid like the metal element.

And finally, we've arrived at **consistency**, the fifth principle, the fire element of the five Ps, the thumb on the fist that pulls it all together.

It's been over two decades since I woke up in royal pain that morning in the county of Kings and was diagnosed with the king's disease. Through all the challenges and changes of life since then, it has been and still is an amazing adventure, and I'm grateful to still be doing my best to stick to my healthy gangsta code.

Consistency consists of two things: discipline and inspiration.

Heavyweight champ Mike Tyson once said that "the worst thing a warrior can lose is his discipline" and that "discipline is doing what you hate to do, but nonetheless doing it like you love it."

I don't know if I would go so far to say it's doing what you hate, 'cause I don't use that word lightly. To me, discipline is consistently taking the necessary actions regardless of how you feel about it. Inspiration is the motivation and influence that compel you to consistently take those actions. When I'm inspired, I feel like I'm supercharged with energy and I can be, do, and have anything I set my mind to and work toward.

The key to my focus for all these years and what has made my healthy lifestyle transformation stick is simply this: I've learned to enjoy the discipline by staying inspired.

Whether on a personal, individual level or in cultures across societies—the meta life skill of consistency is built through structures of what to do (discipline) and models, values, and examples that encourage, empower, and influence you to do it (inspiration).

This is especially true with developing a consistent commitment to healthy living. You know you have to be disciplined about your healthy habits to reap the benefits, but there also has to be something that constantly inspires you to stay on it.

The Power of Change

> I'm not saying I'm gonna change the world, but I
> guarantee that I will spark the brain that will change
> the world.
>
> —*Tupac Shakur*

I believe change is the ultimate inspiration and motivator. We take action because we want to change, or we are forced to change, or because we want to change things. There has to be something you wanna change so badly it inspires and motivates you to move and take the actions necessary, or change happens *to* you, giving you no choice but to change how you're moving and act accordingly.

On the personal level, whether it's a change in perspective, environment, circumstance, or routine, making the right changes and making good choices change things for the good. In human societies, on the social level, I believe change, growth, and progress happen in one of four ways: *riots, reform, revolution, or renaissance*:

A *riot* causes a change in property values and is often really a cry out for a change in policing. It's a temporary inflammation, symptomatic of a chronic social injustice.

A *reform* is a change in a policy. But, in a corrupt system, too often a policy change feels like a slow ambulance bringing a Band-Aid to a gunshot victim.

A *revolution* is a change in power—in theory. But often it's just the players who change, while the game stays the same.

A *renaissance* is a prolific creative period within a popular culture of a people, with profound influence on future generations.

Using my path to well-being as a metaphor, the painful burning eruption of gout I experienced in my twenties made me realize the gross injustice I was doing to myself. It changed what I value; it made me realize my body is my real estate. If I continued to destroy it after being made aware of the cause of the problem, then I would only be devaluing my own property. When my body rioted in the form of gout, I realized the destruction I was causing and I chose to do something about it, make changes, make reforms. My priorities and lifestyle "policies" began shifting from toxic to healing. I reformed my focus from frustration to fitness. Those changes continued to snowball into a full-blown personal revolution that empowered my mind, body, and spirit. By seizing the power of my own choices, I've made revolutionary changes in my life.

All these areas—riots, reforms, and revolutions—on both personal and social levels, do effect change to different degrees, without a doubt, but I wanna zoom in on what a renaissance is and does. From the French language, a renaissance is a rebirth, marking a time of return, renewal, or revival of cultural inspiration in a society. I'll explain how this connects to staying consistent on our well-being journey but hang in there with me as we take a scenic historic route to drive it all home.

The Italian Renaissance

In Italy, their Renaissance was about coming out of the darkness of the Middle Ages into the light of the arts, science, literature, and education as informed by the best of what ancient Greek and Rome had to offer. The invention of the Gutenberg printing press in 1450 allowed leaps in communication throughout Europe through booklets that spread new and exciting ideas that reawakened traditional Greek and Roman culture and values in Italian society. This period was characterized by progressive and influential changes in art, religion, math, science, architecture, and more. Some of the Western world's most renowned thinkers and creatives came out of that inspired period—you know their names: Michelangelo, the sculptor, painter, architect, and poet who sculpted "David"; Niccolò Machiavelli, the guy who inspired 2Pac's alias, Makaveli, was one of the most famous writers of the Italian Renaissance and of history. Galileo was an Italian science giant during the Renaissance who found his true calling in astronomy and physics. He invented his own telescope and verified that the earth does indeed revolve around the sun, and not the other way around as it was widely believed in Europe at the time. Another Italian luminary, Raphael, arguably the greatest painter from this time, painted all the other rooms in the Vatican while Michelangelo was busy with the Sistine Chapel. Another artist, Donatello, was a master sculptor who's also known for his sculpture of David—before Michelangelo made his. It's kinda like Michelangelo bit off of Donatello's David like Ghostface said Biggie's *Ready to Die* album cover bit off Nas's *Illmatic* album cover. But hey, greatness inspires greatness though, right?

And finally, Leonardo da Vinci was a true original Renaissance motherfucker. In fact, he's probably a prototype of what inspired the modern term *Renaissance man*. It's like, what could he *not* do? He was a painter, sculptor, engineer, biologist, and inventor. His sketches and curiosities on human anatomy rendered science in art in ways that still influence both today. But his most famous work— shit, probably the most famous portrait damn near ever—is the *Mona Lisa*. It's been called the best known, the most visited, the most written about, the most sung about, the most parodied work of art in the world. Even master hip-hop storyteller Slick Rick wrote a "Mona Lisa" joint inspired by the iconic artwork. Now, I still to this day don't know who in the hell Mona Lisa was, but I know Leonardo da Vinci made her ass hella famous.

The renaissance facilitated a boom in interest in the body, anatomy, biology, health, and physical education. The concentration of all that talent and influence from one period is crazy, right? But of course, Europe ain't got no monopoly on greatness or renaissance periods.

Next stop: Harlem.

The Harlem Renaissance

In the 1900s, millions of Black folks left the segregated South for what they felt was a lesser of two evils for a better life in the North, and many ended up relocating to Manhattan's Harlem neighborhood. Believe it or not, the area was originally developed as a residential spot for well-to-do white families, but once Black families started moving into the vacant spaces, as the saying goes—there goes the neighborhood! This small mile-and-a-half chunk of Upper Manhattan, named after a Dutch city in the Netherlands (Haarlem), and mostly occupied by Italian and Jewish communities prior to the great Black Southern exodus, became a haven for Black Southern refugees, which soon blossomed into a major cultural mecca.

The Harlem Renaissance helped Black writers, artists, and activists be more in control of the representation of Black identity, and it provided an authentic inspiring account of the multidimensional beauty of Blackness at a time when it was still illegal for a Black person to drink from the same water fountain as a white person. This "golden age" in Harlem didn't last hundreds of years like the Italian Renaissance did; in fact, from its beginning to its peak and then decline, the Harlem Renaissance lasted just under two decades, but its undeniable legacy and influence have deeply impacted the worlds of art, music, literature, theater, social justice, modern Black culture, and so much more, and continue to do so decades after its heyday. It's one of the most important, impactful, and enduring cultural movements America has ever seen.

Some of the most notable dynamic luminaries that emerged out of the fertile Nile of the Harlem Renaissance were writer, poet, and playwright Langston Hughes; author, playwright, and filmmaker Zora

Neale Hurston; iconic trumpeter Louis Armstrong; Billie Holiday; and many, many others.

Like I mentioned, most research you find will tell you that the Harlem Renaissance grew out of two things: the great migration and the thousands of industrial jobs made available by the demands of America's World War I war machine. While it is true that a large number of Black folks moved to the North and congregated in NYC, and it's also true that World War I created a lot of jobs in industries that supported the war and those northern-based jobs attracted lots of Black folks to the area, these two things alone can't be what caused the Renaissance—groups of people migrate and work industrial jobs all the time and no major Renaissance necessarily just pops out of it. So, what was the cause, the inspiration behind the Harlem Renaissance? Why that community?

Consider this: Those folks must have had to be tremendously inspired by something for a Renaissance to sprout out of those conditions and circumstances at a time when being Black in the US was the equivalent to being legally considered a second-class citizen or worse. And at the same time, this community had to somehow have access to the means of production to be able to reproduce and magnify and celebrate their cultural enthusiasm on such a phenomenal scale.

What caused that wave of inspiration to rise in such a powerful and prolific way?

In the same way that the Italian Renaissance drew its inspiration from its historical roots in Rome and Greece, the Harlem Renaissance drew its inspiration from ancient roots too, but of the African-descended roots of its community.

Harlem was home to the Jamaica-born political activist, publisher, journalist, entrepreneur, and orator, the Honorable Marcus Garvey and was the heart and base of his operations in the 1920s from which he successfully recruited millions of members around the diaspora into the largest Black power organization ever assembled—the United

Negro Improvement Association. The Hannibal of his era, Garvey raised up the red, black, and green flag of African liberation and ignited the Harlem scene and beyond with his empowering vision of a free, united, and self-sufficient Black world of possibilities. His motivating message and movement spread like a wildfire and lit up the hearts and minds of all those relocated refugees and underdogs in the process. Soon, the Harlem-based UNIA had opened seven hundred branches all across the country, and they eventually established international chapters on three continents and in the Caribbean.

Garvey's African-centered empowerment philosophy instilled a sense of Black pride that inspired and incited the Harlem Renaissance in a way that cannot be overstated. His dream of Black power, Black excellence, and Black well-being was a powerful river that flooded the Harlem Renaissance with inspiration. The enduring legacy of the Harlem Renaissance continues to send ripple effects in Black culture and world culture.

When it comes to inspiration through the arts, popular Renaissance movements are unlike any other force. That early Harlem energy carried over into generation after generation and saw the likes of people's champions like Malcolm X join its ranks and expand the impact of Harlem's legacy to even higher heights. There's something powerful that stirs when whole swells of passionate creative voices and charismatic people start to gravitate toward a common cultural pulse. One of my favorite OG groups of all times is The Last Poets. They were popular in the early '70s, but they carried on the energy of the Harlem Renaissance like no other poetry groups have done since. These brothers wrote and spoke their unapologetic poetics the rousing rhythms of African drumming on street corners and in alleyways and pool halls—spreading the seeds of rhythm and poetry that influenced icons like Gil Scott-Heron and made those guys the forefathers of rap.

Enter hip-hop.

The Natural Birth of Rap

The word "rap" was used as a slang term in the early '70s. It meant conversing, speaking, or talking with someone. Cats would say, "Hey, let me rap at ya" when they wanted to talk to you about something important, personal, or interesting. H. Rap Brown, former chairman of the Student Nonviolent Coordinating Committee (SNCC) and later the minister of justice for the Black Panther Party, talked about rap in his autobiography released in 1969. He said his sharp rhyme tongue playing the dozens and other word and rhyme games earned him the nickname Rap as a youngster. Later, H. Rap Brown (now known as Jamil al-Amin) was renowned for his ability to lay down a heavy political rap and speak in a way that got cats thinking about changing their social conditions for the better.

By the time the man credited by many respected pioneers within the culture as the founding father of hip-hop, the muscular-framed, Jamaican-born DJ Kool Herc, was spinning records in the 1970s, powered by lamp-posts in the Bronx on Sedgwick and Cedar Avenues, the streets were more than ready for all that legendary momentum from the Harlem Renaissance and the revolutionary '60s to explode into a new phenomenon. An exciting mash-up of music, dance, poetry, art, and culture that would soon do what the Harlem Renaissance did, but in spades around the world.

Hip-hop hit the scene like Tyson hit boxing. It was young, hungry, powerful, electrifying. Early pioneers like Grandmaster Flash and the Furious Five, KRS-One, among others, stood out from the pack to me because they carried on the spirit of speaking our truths and experiences and bringing light to the culture on a level of the high bar set by the great orators and poets and teachers before them.

When my older brother Troy first introduced me to hip-hop, he assigned me the task of becoming an emcee.

He said, "I'mma be the DJ and you gon' be the emcee."

And from the first day he called me that, it became my calling.

The Other Renaissance of the '80s

During the golden era of the '80s, when hip-hop was manifesting itself through the culture of spray painting, pop locking, back spinning, and party rocking; with hit films like *Wild Style*, *Beat Street*, *Breakin'*, and *Krush Groove;* and classic artists like Kurtis Blow, Run-D.M.C., Beastie Boys, Doug E. Fresh, Slick Rick, LL Cool J, Biz Markie, Big Daddy Kane, Eric B. & Rakim, EPMD, MC Lyte, BDP, De La Soul, Public Enemy, Ice-T, N.W.A., and many more; there was also another contagious cultural wave happening at the same time: *the fitness boom.*

If you're not too young, you probably remember the sweatbands, leg warmers, and leotards that characterized the aerobic fitness explosion of the '80s, but it was happening side by side with hip-hop's popular surge, and it definitely influenced hip-hop's style and vice versa. Aerobic workouts incorporated popular dance music and involved running, stretching, and other group calisthenics routines.

Aerobics-style workouts were first developed by an Air Force surgeon and exercise physiologist, Dr. Kenneth Cooper, and Colonel Pauline Potts, a physical therapist, but it was actress Jane Fonda's exercise videos in 1982 that blew the fitness craze up in mainstream culture. You can see a clear example of that aerobic leotard and headband fusion with the urban fashion of the time in the hip-hop cult classic film series *Breakin'* that dropped in 1984. The exercise and entertainment industries were recognizing the talents and skills of b-boys and girls and they in turn were influencing modern trends in exercise dance and fitness. Hip-hop dance culture and aerobic dance culture sampled and shaped each other with global results.

Recreational running had already become a huge phenomenon in the '70s and continued to gain momentum in the '80s as well. The same Dr. Cooper who pioneered aerobics and saw aerobic activity as the cornerstone of physical fitness had created a cardiovascular fitness test consisting of a one-and-a-half-mile run, done in under twelve minutes, which inspired the standard used in military training. The research and ideas he brought forth were endorsed by the mainstream medical community in the early 1970s, and his ideas helped running get its footing as a huge recreational fitness trend of that period. Fitness was in the air.

The mega success of sports-drama films like *The Karate Kid* and *Rocky* also fanned the flames of working out in pop culture during the '80s. Actors Ralph Macchio and Sylvester Stallone became not only pop icons, but also through their roles as Daniel-san and Rocky Balboa, they became enduring cult symbols for the virtues of sport. Karate-school and boxing-gym attendance surged during the '80s largely because of how these films used art to inspire an appreciation for karate and boxing. Fitness culture, urban culture, and hip-hop culture skyrocketed alongside one another during those golden years.

BREAKING

I remember back in the '80s how we used to press play on the boom box, break out the cardboard or linoleum scraps, and practice our break-dance moves all day and night. As a young, aspiring hip-hop artist, dancing was a part of my performances and also just a fun hobby I enjoyed doing with the homies. We created coordinated dance routines, worked on stretching for splits, and put in hours and hours of work every day. At the time, I never really thought of it as exercise or working out, but the athleticism of break dancing (breaking) was actually a very healthy form of fitness training. But it wasn't in any of those official boxes. There was no school but the streets for spinning on your head. It was our kung fu. It was our yoga. It was our capoeira. Even popping and locking, when I look back at it, was kind of like tai chi.

Doing those moves required energy, flexibility, strength, and endurance. It was super challenging, but it was fun and exciting and inclusive. It didn't matter who you were or what you had, if you were into breaking you felt like you belonged to a scene, you were down with a thriving cultural movement. From their early origins in the late '70s and early '80s, hip-hop and the wide-ranging world of health, fitness, and wellness have had a lot of meaningful chemistry and connections.

Return of Inspiration

At this time in the '80s, you had this really interesting cross-pollination dynamic going on between this fresh, new positive culture among the youth happening simultaneously alongside the running and aerobic fitness boom of the '70s and '80s and then, bam—the CIA's devastating crack agenda comes along and changes the narrative and the values of the culture in a negative downward spiral.

Drug rap, cocaine music, gangster rap, trap music took over the airwaves, on one hand giving a much-needed voice to the streets but then, at the same time, in many ways negatively influencing the hearts and minds of the youth. What had been, for the most part, a culture of peace, love, unity, and having fun became a culture criticized for its misogyny, violence, capitalistic ethos, and celebrated drug abuse.

Still, over the years, the business of being a hip-hop artist has offered practical and progressive benefits (though the overall capitalistic ideas are problematic); hip-hop has become the global pop culture across international borders, influencing many cultures around the world. Artists like Jay-Z and Ye cracked the safe so well they became rap's first billionaires, leveraging their phenomenal musical instincts and skills, cultural influence, and business acumen. Hip-hop is on the *Forbes* list, it's in all the Hollywood blockbusters, it's even at the top of the gospel charts, R&B charts, and pop charts; it's off the charts.

With all this in mind, I believe there is a Renaissance happening right now.

The waves of art inspiration and health and fitness have been ebbing and flowing since the pharaohs were commissioning artwork depicting their Heb-Sed festivals, where the king would have to demonstrate his physical fitness through running and other feats of strength every so often to maintain his eligibility to lead. The saying *ankh, udja, seneb* (life, prosperity, health) was a national greeting of ancient Egypt in the time of the pharaohs.

There's a cyclical, cosmic pattern at work in everything. From the universal level down to the atomic and quantum levels, the waves of the past continue to reverberate onto the shores of the present and ripple into the future. These oscillating patterns and polyrhythms give life, in all of its vast complexities, its predictability, consistency, routine, and balance. Life persists. Decomposition produces regeneration. History repeats itself. Things come back around.

In our current era, when the wellness industry has grown to a four-trillion-dollar valuation, coupled with hip-hop's global influence and commercial success and the resurgence of health and fitness in pop culture in the aftermath of a pandemic, I believe the next big wave is shaping up to be an urban holistic renaissance.

I promised you I'd tie all this back into staying consistent on our well-being journey, and I hope you're still with me. I'm putting forth the vision that we have an opportunity to play our parts in a new uprising at its beginning. It's much more than a short-term fad or trend. We're in a period that holds the potential for a new renaissance, a time of revival, an age of enlightenment, a new golden era. I believe we are at the convergence of two great movements: the global influence hip-hop and the holistic industry of well-being.

The Age of the "Wellionaires"

Even from hip-hop's beginnings in the '70s and '80s, rappers like Melle Mel and LL Cool J made us want to be strong and swole because of their fit physiques and stamina onstage. Songs like Kool Moe Dee's "Go See the Doctor" and KRS-One's "Beef" and "My Philosophy," and even the posse track "Self Destruction" expressed hip-hop's ability to creatively speak to issues that affect our health and well-being. Sports figures from basketball to boxing have long embraced hip-hop culture in their attitude and swag. Here are some recent examples, just a slice of how hip-hop and health, fitness, and wellness are exploring alignment more than ever:

- West-Coast lyricist The Game leads a yearly fitness boot camp called 60 Days of Fitness.
- Method Man has his own athletic training and cannabis brand—Tical Athletics.
- Jim Jones reps his crew's own fitness brand, VampFitt, and he and other New York rappers collectively promote their weight lifting comradery to millions of their social-media followers.
- E.D.I. of the Outlawz, Lil Fame of M.O.P., Killer Mike, Scarface, David Banner, Fat Joe, Timbaland, and countless other rappers have had huge weight-loss transformations.
- Houston rapper Slim Thug has his own fitness brand, called HuslFit.
- Urban calisthenics crews like the Bartendaz out of Harlem and others around the globe train in the parks and gyms to hip-hop music, mentoring youth and promoting mental and physical fitness in their hoods. In my opinion, these calisthenics crews are like a new, modern expression of b-boy and b-girl culture.
- Rapper and actor Will Smith is promoting the fitness apparel brand Bel-Air Athletics, inspired by his iconic TV show.

- His son Jaden Smith started a vegan food truck initiative for the homeless. He also launched Just Water, a progressive, sustainable water company.

- Rick Ross—yes, the heavyweight chicken-wing king himself—even has his own fitness brand, RossFit. Despite the Wingstop franchises he owns, Rick Ross has spoken often about his commitment to improving his own health after experiencing several seizures over the years.

- Being the meditating, rapping, Beats-headphones-rocking, world-class baller he is, LeBron James's love for hip-hop and what it brings to his game in terms of inspiration is well known. King James is constantly tapping into hip-hop music. James and RZA partnered with Calm, one of the largest meditation apps in the industry.

- In the '90s, the Wu Tang Clan revitalized interest in martial arts within hip-hop culture. Among many ventures since, RZA and other Wu-Tang members have partnered with PETA. RZA also aligned with the tea brand Tazo to lead insightful meditation retreats.

- The Chicago-born, Grammy award–winning rapper Lupe Fiasco holds a black belt in martial arts. His docuseries *Beat N' Path* follows Lupe on a cross-cultural journey to China where he practices kung fu with Chinese masters in the mountains and explores China's hip-hop scene.

- Wiz Khalifa is a passionate martial artist and MMA fan who has gotten his weight up over the years as a student of jujitsu and Muay Thai. He shares clips of his morning training sessions daily on his Instagram to millions of followers. He was an early investor and partner in the MMA's Professional Fighters League, a rising organization that promotes MMA with a unique, seasonal format with playoffs, finals, and million-dollar prizes for the champion of each weight class.

- For years, Snoop Dogg has been outspoken about his interest in plant-based foods. Snoop made many investments in plant-based opportunities. He explained in *Forbes* back in 2020 that he decided to change his diet to improve his overall health; he was even an early investor in Beyond Meat. He has said that when he introduced his family to Beyond Meat, he snuck it in without telling them and nobody noticed the difference.

- There are plenty of vegan rappers and entrepreneurs that are killin' it and who have been on it for years before it was as popular as it is today, like my homies DJ Cavem, Super Nova Slom, Grey of Plant Based Drippin, and many others. Styles P of the rap group The Lox and his wife own a franchise of juice bars and a natural-supplements company in different inner-city neighborhoods in New York City. Drill-rap icon NLE Choppa converted to veganism and has become a very outspoken advocate for conscious, healthy living.

- Although he's not vegan, Jay-Z's support of plant-based living has put his money where his mouth is. Jigga man has invested in more than a couple plant-based companies and campaigns. He cofounded 22 Days Nutrition, the vegan meal-planning service, with his wife, Beyoncé, and exercise physiologist Marco Borges. In the foreword to Borges's book, *The Greenprint: Plant-Based Diet, Best Body, Better World,* they wrote, "We used to think of health as a diet—some worked for us, some didn't. Once we looked at health as the truth, instead of a diet, it became a mission for us to share that truth and lifestyle with as many people as possible."

Even yoga has been influenced by the urban wave (and vice versa). When you think about yoga, you might think of zen'd out, relaxing, new-age-sounding music, but hip-hop is getting its namaste on, too.

Rapper Mc Yogi has been single-handedly holding down hip-hop in the yoga space for years. You may not have heard of him, but his consistent focus has made him a mainstay of some of the biggest yoga festivals in the world.

When artist Janelle Monáe dropped her hit single, "Yoga," it turned up urban interest in yoga around the country. Today, yoga is more popular than ever in urban communities. Britteny Floyd-Mayo created what she calls the "Trap Yoga" experience. It's a vinyasa-style yoga workout, performed to trap music and accompanied by her inspirational, equal-parts pep-talk and real-talk "ratchet affirmations." She was inspired to create Trap Yoga because she didn't feel culturally connected to the "thin, upper-class white girl" vibe that is typical of many yoga spaces in the US.

Hip-hop is even tapping into the mental-health space as well. Cohost of one of the biggest hip-hop talk platforms, *The Breakfast Club*, Charlamagne tha God invested in the world's first mental-health gym. His *Breakfast Club* cohost Angela Yee opened her own juice bars. Big Sean's raps are laced with mental health–related and self-care bars. Gucci Mane's radical mental and physical fitness transformation as told in his best-selling autobiography has inspired millions.

There is no place you can go in the modern urban world—whether it be sports, fitness, or well-being—that isn't weaved together in some way or another with hip-hop. And it's growing every day in every way.

We are definitely at the dawn of an urban holistic Renaissance. And I'm so inspired by it. Do you see where this Wellionaires wave is going?

HIP-HOP IS A MIND-SET, A FORCE, A SPIRIT, AND
ATTITUDE.

—THE CULTURE

When the Culture Is Well-Being

> When we move, the whole world follows in our path.
>
> —*Common*

When our personal, social, and spiritual practices are based on a high standard of holistic, healthy living, we have a culture that reinforces well-being. We celebrate what nourishes us. We popularize what heals us. We value what inspires healthy living. We are committed to nourishing and flourishing as individuals, families, and communities. We invest in wellness as a society. Art inspires well-being. Literature inspires well-being. Science supports well-being. Educational institutions support well-being. Industry, activism, architecture, city planning, every aspect of our collective will is about the business of well-being.

When motivation comes in social waves it's easy to get inspired and take advantage of the positive momentum all around you; though I believe the most important and most sustainable way to stay inspired comes from kindling our own inner light. It's so helpful when we can light our candle and multiply our fire off the inspiration of others.

To me there is no doubt that fusions between hip-hop and wellness are the future, and I believe as a community we each have a powerful part to play in it—as visionaries, owners, enthusiasts, investors, and creatives.

As sure as every superhero needs a theme song, every uprising needs a soundtrack. One of my personal missions as an artist and songwriter over the last ten years has been creating that healthy gangsta soundtrack.

I call it "fit-hop."

CHAPTER 16

Tao of Fit-Hop

You want to be strong, but you want to have that strength last. The way that you get in the game and stay on top of your game is to be consistent.... The workout is never over.

—*Grandmaster Melle Mel*

You can view the phases and periods of our lives like the developing and hatching of eggs. These various periods provide us with protective "shells" that we are nourished by and grow in.

Inside these shells, those walls of limited understanding protect, guide, and feed us as we mature in that space of thoughts, beliefs, and behaviors until the inevitable cracks start to appear.

All the shells we find ourselves in can protect us for a while. But once we start to outgrow that shell, it starts to crack from the pressure. Then we get curious about the new light that is shining in on us.

Sometimes, this light seems blinding, especially when we are used to living in the comfortable darkness of our familiar shell. What once was a safe and comfortable space that facilitated your nourishment and growth becomes, over time, inadequate to sustain your growth and development. Once the time has come, if you don't get out of that egg, it will become your casket.

There are certain "eggs" of understanding that we find ourselves being nourished by, but we also have to know when it's time to crack that shell and let the light in. There is a time when you've outgrown your shell and there is more of the world waiting for you to explore in new ways. This is a necessary and natural part of our continuous growth and development.

Even your physical life itself, your meat suit, is but a temporary egg where our spirits grow and develop until they are ready to hatch into the even greater beyond in the mystery of existence.

Growing, hatching, transcending: that's the pattern I see that we are all a part of.

The personal revolution I experienced through health and fitness inspired me to reevaluate my values and helped lead me where I wanted to go next with my music career. Artistically, I needed a change. Not all, but the majority of the music I'd created with dead prez over the years had been about problems and issues that we as a community are suffering or battling or fighting against—the public school system, the police state, the prison industrial complex, the negative effects of drug abuse, economic oppression, racist and classist treatment under unjust power structures, etc. It was real music, but it was heavy stuff. That emotional weight is a lot to carry. I had grown a lot over time, and I knew I wanted to incorporate more of a positive balance to the legacy of songs that I'm leaving behind, and at a point I realized I had outgrown many of the pessimistic perspectives I had been so passionate about in my teens. Don't get it twisted, I'm still and always will be RBG for life, but some of the sentiments I held had become a drain on my spirit instead of feeding it. Healthy living had given me a much more positive and proactive outlook on life, and I wanted my music to express and accentuate that more often. I came to realize that I needed to focus on more of what I'm for than what I'm against. After cracking the shell of my earlier dead prez career, something new emerged.

Often as artists (and as people in general) when we feel we're in the dark about what to do next, just in time, like an egg about to hatch, the light comes in.

Serendipity

As serendipity would have it, I was sitting on a chair in the comfort of the then chocolate-brown walls of my home studio, just sitting around staring at the Bruce Lee and Muhammad Ali posters, Buddhas, and other eclectic whatnots sprawled around, hoping that showing up in front of my equipment with a willingness to work would make me worthy and lucky enough to be hit with a creative lightning bolt that would be musically productive.

On my wooden altar in the corner, I had an eight-by-ten vintage photograph of my late maternal granddad, Mr. Benny Frank, that my mom had framed and gifted to me. My granddad's photo sat next to a green and healthy aloe plant that I nicknamed Serendipity.

I had only heard Oprah Winfrey using that word; she said it's "important to leave room for serendipity," but I didn't know what it meant exactly; it just sounded like a magical kind of word to me. So, I looked up the definition: "Serendipity: the occurrence and development of events by chance in a happy or beneficial way."

I thought, Wow, how many times has serendipity been happening in my life and I didn't fully acknowledge it? So many great things have happened in spite of all the hardships, and I'd been so focused on my struggles that I hadn't really developed my gratitude-awareness muscle enough to recognize how blessed I'd been as well.

I was once homeless but got signed and made a global impact as an emcee.

I'd been incarcerated but it was a catalyst to getting more focused in my mind about my vision for my life.

I'd been sick with gout, but it put me in a position to appreciate and take much better care of myself.

I'd broken boards and run marathons on the same foot that was once crippled by poor lifestyle choices.

Blessings often come disguised as challenges. Serendipity had been happening all my life and I was starting to see my life through the lens of gratitude. Something about that word spoke to me deeply, almost as if once I heard it, it was a secret word that revealed new magical possibilities, miracles even, in my life.

Word-sound power is real. I resonated with the word serendipity so much so that as I mentioned earlier, I named the aloe plant on my altar Serendipity to help the serendipity continue to flourish and be viable in my life.

My granddaddy, Serendipity, and I would sit in the creative lab together for hours at a time.

On this particularly serendipitous day I had cooked up a drum sequence and I thought the loop had some promise to it. I set the tempo to ninety-five beats per minute, which I had figured out over the years was my natural go-to tempo as an emcee.

As I was accustomed to doing in the studio as part of my creative process, I let the drums just knock on repeat over and over and over until it became so monotonous that I kind of slipped into a mild trance.

That day, it seemed like my grandfather's energy started speaking to me. It felt like his presence was actually in the room giving me suggestions. It's not like I heard his actual voice in the room externally, but it's more like I felt his energy making suggestions in my heart and mind.

The idea arose: "Make a song about running."

I don't know why, but it felt like my granddad had whispered it in my ear.

"Wait a minute," I thought, "where is that idea coming from?" and "Yo, a song about running? That might be kinda dope."

I started listening to the drums more, allowing my inner ear to tune into what I felt like the song needed next. I started feeling a calling to certain ambient sounds in my head and I started seeing images of Kenyan runners in a field in my mind.

Fingering my keyboard for melodic nuggets, I selected an ambient midi sound from my digital sound bank and improvised some notes until a simple melody surfaced that felt right at home with the drums, so I looped it.

Then I had this open ambient groove just pulsing on repeat and all my attention was just locked into the vibe.

I pulled up some YouTube footage of Kenyan runners and muted the video sound and turned up my track while watching the images of the Kenyan landscape to inspire what would fit next. Watching the runners training in the hills with my beat as the soundtrack felt magical.

I could see all kinds of visuals and the visuals started to come out in pieces of lyrics and melodic couplets.

Before long I was harmonizing a vocal melody with the phrase "This life is a journey, some are going, some are coming…" and it sounded like it could be a good start for the chorus.

I sat there in the studio for maybe hours, just in a creative flow state. Ideas were flooding so fast that I needed to step away from the studio environment and get a handle on it all. My creative downloads be heavy. I was being flooded with a creative downpour.

While watching the Kenyans running, it dawned on me to bounce a copy of the beat and test it out on an actual run and see what kind of spontaneous lyrics might come up during it.

The results of that process became the song "Runner's High" and that creative inspiration led to a whole new approach to hip-hop for me.

A journey of a thousand miles begins one step at a time
I refuse to sit back on the side and let life keep passing me by
Pushing forward at a comfortable pace, the race is not for
    the swift I just take it in stride
Both feet on the ground, but it feel like I'm touching the sky
No drug in my veins
I got a runner's high

                        —"Runner's High"

In the following four weeks, I produced, wrote, and recorded thirteen more joints about martial-arts training, gym life, yoga, sobriety, plant-based eating, lifting weights, everything under the sun from my healthy lifestyle and fitness experiences, and these fourteen joints would become the world's first ever "fit-hop" album, *The Workout*.

Besides being an album centered in health and fitness, the project is also unique for a hip-hop album because it has no profanity, not even the N-word. I decided to make all the lyrics family appropriate in honor of a request from one of my late OGs, Baba Jim, who is featured as the drill-sergeant voice on the song "Joe Louis." Baba Jim was my son Twezo's teacher from pre-K to fifth grade at a private Afrikan boys' warrior shule called Sankofa. Baba Jim didn't like much hip-hop but he was a fan of my music. He was not a yes-man about *anything*. Baba Jim was a hardcore ex-Marine and as direct and in-your-face as they come. He suggested to me not long before he transitioned that I should leave out the cursing so that more families could enjoy my music. Since he was going to be featured on the *Workout* album I agreed, and leaving the profanity out became a signature part of my approach to this new "fit-hop" expression, in his honor.

We've lost so many rappers to the culture of violence; it plagues not only the entertainment industry but also the community that inspires it. Do you think Biggie Smalls knew what was coming when he named his album *Ready to Die*? Do you think 'Pac really saw his own death around the corner? Our words matter. Our lives matter. And what we tell ourselves matters. But keeping it all the way one hundred, we have lost even more hip-hop artists to health issues and poor diets than pistols. If dead prez's body of music expresses the call for social justice through a political revolution, fit-hop expresses the call to action for elevating personal and community health.

And of course, it's all connected.

A Tool for Inspiration

I coined the term "fit-hop" as a simple way to distinguish this new style, but the focus is not just about physical fitness, it's also about the health and well-being of mind, body, and spirit—360 degrees of fitness. It's a subgenre of hip-hop that combines profanity-free, hard-hitting hip-hop music with non-preachy, healthy lifestyle song concepts to enhance workouts, increase endorphins, and inspire holistic well-being and fitness.

I was already experimenting with precursors for "fit-hop" from the beginning of dead prez's career. We made a demo with Lord Jamar called "Learn Karate" that was never released. On dead prez's debut album *Let's Get Free* we dropped the vegan anthem "Be Healthy," and on our sophomore follow-up *RBG: Revolutionary but Gangsta,* we featured the training anthems "Way of Life" and "50 in the Clip." But when serendipity whispered "runner's high" into my ear, I fully realized fit-hop was *its own thing* and that I was to be its vehicle.

Jeet kune do was Bruce Lee's personal expression of the martial arts, and fit-hop is my personal musical expression of hip-hop and healthy living. With fit-hop, I found my creative mojo again. I found new inspiration. I found the direction that my music can continue to evolve in moving forward.

My creative process for fit-hop is inspired by my huge admiration for the sport of boxing and martial arts.

With fit-hop, I try to have fun and bring the spirit of sport to my songwriting process. I imagine that working on fit-hop joints in the studio is a metaphor for a fighter training in the gym. I like to have a "champ camp" kind of mentality while I'm creating the albums. I'm eating a certain way to keep my mind clear; I'm listening to certain things like podcasts or audiobooks to keep me motivated and inspired like a fighter being encouraged by his cornerman. I'm running consistently, doing lots of roadwork and calisthenics to keep my fitness up and my spirit charged. My jabs are my bars, my hooks are my choruses. I get my "lyrical cardio" recording multiple takes and demos until I memorize the verses and can say the final take from memory without reading them off my notes. I'm working on the song elements and arrangements like a fight team develops a winning strategy for their fighter to execute. Sparring is the collaboration with other artists and feedback I get along the way for making adjustments and edits. Arriving at mixing the finished album is like the feeling of showing up for the championship fight you've been training for. You've put in the work and all those rounds of the mixing process are when you and the team bring it all together for the world to experience!

Ain't no studio healthy gangsta. Real-life training—mentally, physically, and spiritually—and authentically living a healthy and holistic lifestyle are essential for the craftsmanship of the sound and songs. You have to live it to give it.

I am super inspired by the vintage, gritty aesthetics of those old-school hole-in-the-wall kind of gyms, and that's a big part of the inspiration behind the grainy, black-and-white styling and art direction for my fit-hop albums. I'm always tapping into Ali, Bruce Lee, and many others for new creative revelations and ways to incorporate my admiration for them into what I do.

RBG FIT CLUB: The Vision

I'm invested in fit-hop as a tool of inspiration and as a form of *artivism*. I believe we have to be the change we wanna see. Fit-hop started as my own personal expression, but I want to help other artists find their voice and sound in fit-hop as well; that way it can spread and multiply for generations to come. Imagine a day when fit-hop music and culture will have its own legion of creatives trailblazing on the cultural and creative sides, and at the same time owning and benefiting from the business and growth potentials involved as well. Like hip-hop, fit-hop is bigger than just the music. I see fit-hop as the catchword for infinite possibilities between hip-hop and wellness—from products and services to events and experiences, to entertainment and education. The sky's the limit.

When I got the idea to create *The Workout*, the RBG FIT CLUB brand was born right alongside it because I wanted to also expand my platform for promoting healthy living beyond music. Part of staying consistent is accountability, and ain't nothing like starting a movement to hold yourself accountable. I didn't want to be the rapper that used to be on healthy shit and fell off, I wanted to stay inspired. Inspiring others keeps me inspired with a higher purpose, and RBG FIT CLUB is a way to hold myself accountable in order to do that. The aim of the brand is to be an identity that folks on the same frequency can recognize and feel a connection to. I based the brand philosophy on five major life lessons that I learned on my wellness journey—the five principles we've spent time with through this book: knowledge, nutrition, exercise, rest, and consistency.

The Bird and the Bar

For RBG FIT CLUB's logo, I wanted to come up with something that represents "reaching bigger goals." Drawing on inspiration from ancient Egypt, I chose Heru the falcon for a few reasons. With eyesight eight times more accurate than a human, the falcon represents higher vision. It also symbolizes the choice to rise up to the level of your higher self. With its powerful speed and strength as a hunter, the falcon's ability to fly high and swoop down on its prey at over two hundred miles per hour makes it a great metaphor of strength, upliftment, and vision.

I reached out to my homey, the legendary art director Shannon Washington of Swash Creative, and told her I wanted to create something timeless. I asked her to cook up a logo using the Heru glyph and I had her add an iron barbell in the talons—symbolizing my vision for raising the bar on health and fitness in our culture. She developed what became our official "wings-up" emblem.

With the logo, and with the brand as a whole, my aim was also to help raise the vibration of the definition of fitness from just being focused on physical strength, endurance, flexibility, and vitality but to also include the mind and spirit as a whole. Baked into the fabric of the RBG FIT CLUB brand is a belief that an authentic, healthy lifestyle is unique for each person and that we should take a custom-fit approach that "fits" our own needs and circumstances. That's why I didn't decide to start with a physical gym space; I want to encourage you to understand that you are your own gym. RBG FIT CLUB is a mindset and a way of being. It's a gym without ceilings or walls. Membership for this gym is about living the five Ps in your own way. That's why our mantra is *membership is living it.*

The RBG FIT CLUB signature brand colors are yellow and black, inspired by the yellow-and-black tracksuit that my hero Bruce Lee made iconic in *Game of Death*, the last film he was working on before his transition.

I was just channeling and pulling inspiration from meaningful elements of my health and fitness journey.

RBG FIT CLUB is for the culture and brings everything I'm for and about under one accord—it is family owned and operated; the dues are the lifestyle. Membership ain't about paying no fees, it's about living the five Ps. It's rooted in the well-being of the community, and it's bigger than hip-hop!

CHAPTER 17

Living It

On a sunny Saturday in 2022, Lester Wright, a Black World War II vet and lifelong runner who just happened to be—get this—one hundred years old at the time, ran the one hundred–meter dash in the senior masters division at the Penn Relays. But not only did Mr. Lester Wright run, a feat in itself at a century old, he set a world record for his age group finishing in only 26.34 seconds!

Keep going is the mantra.

Another one-hundred-years-young runner, Fauja Singh, became the first one-hundred-year-old to finish a marathon in 2011! He completed the Toronto Waterfront Marathon, running 26.2 miles in eight hours, twenty-five minutes, and seventeen seconds.

Keep going is the mantra.

Baltimore's Keith "Running Man" Boissiere, a Trinidad-and-Tobago native nearing his seventies, made headlines and even landed a sponsorship deal because of his status as a local legend for consistently completing epic twenty-mile jogs across the city—not once in a while, but daily! Even though he was diagnosed with stage-four chronic kidney disease in his late thirties, he never let that stop him. His doctor told him that running would help him maintain his health and he's been running for his life ever since—logging twenty miles almost every single day for over thirty years, through rain, sleet, or snow.

Keep going is the mantra.

Miss Ida Keeling lived to the ripe old age of 106. She was a competitive track-and-field athlete who didn't get started running until she was sixty-seven. She was coached by her daughter and went on to run and compete for the rest of her life. In her inspirational book, *Can't Nothing Bring Me Down*, Miss Ida said that her secret to health and fitness was working out two to four times a week and dancing. She ate greens, fruit, and cod-liver oil consistently and, being the healthy gangsta she was, she also treated herself to cognac with her coffee once a week. She holds masters records in the sixty-meter and the hundred-meter distances for women in both the ninety-five to ninety-nine and hundred-plus age groups.

Keep going is the mantra.

I like stories like these because they keep me inspired on my own health and fitness journey as I age. Keep going is my mantra, and when I see examples like these, I know that a long and healthy life is possible if I just keep putting in the work.

Achieving Consistency

The key to long-term success in any endeavor is to identify the principles that lead to success and work those principles. As far as healthy living, the five principles have kept me healthy for the last twenty-plus years. Mindset, diet, fitness, relaxation practices, and staying enthusiastic about maintaining wellness all work together as a health-promoting, fitness-developing, and vitality-enhancing lifestyle.

It's been said that 80 percent of success in anything is mindset and 20 percent is mechanics. You have to be in the right frame of mind to succeed no matter what it is you're doing. Your psychology has to be in support of and in sync with what the vision and mission is. Another way to break that eighty-twenty ratio down is to flip it and look at it like this: if the eighty-twenty principle holds true, that means one of the five Ps is responsible for 80 percent of the results.

Of the four principles we've delved into so far in this book—from knowledge to nutrition to exercise to rest—the most important one, the one that ties it all together and helps you stay on it and reap the benefits of these principles long-term, is the principle of consistency. Let's remember that consistency is achieved by two things: discipline and inspiration.

Enjoy the Discipline

You won't always feel motivated. That's why we have to learn to be disciplined.

We achieve that by committing to routines and rituals and regimens that provide guides, structure, and accountability for us to take action whether we feel like it or not, because we've already decided it's in our best interest and made the commitment to follow through regardless of how we might feel. There're memes floating around on social media that will tell you motivation is bullshit; you just need to get off your ass and be disciplined. While I understand the sentiment, I disagree with the premise. Discipline is the action, but you need the motivation behind the action to stay consistent over time.

We're not discipline machines. We don't just run off meaningless commands. Our willpower is fueled by inspiration. When you are inspired you are more likely to stay disciplined. So, it's not about sitting around and waiting on inspiration to hit you randomly and inconsistently. It's about knowing how to generate, channel, and harness your inspiration consistently, so you are able to enjoy the discipline and reap the benefits for the long run. If you stay inspired, you'll be able to enjoy the discipline; and in order to stay disciplined you need to learn how to stay inspired.

That's what this final chapter is all about: developing your strategy to stay consistent and disciplined by understanding how to stay inspired and motivated and consistently take action for your well-being.

A Way of Life

As I said, if you had to choose the one principle of the five that would give you the most bang for your buck it would hands down be *consistency*. Without consistency, the benefits of the other principles can't even be activated, much less maintained. Consistency is really about how true you wanna be to this shit. How well do you wanna feel and live? What level of health do you wanna experience? Being consistent is about finding that groove, riding the waves, falling off and getting back to it, and staying on it. It's about making health and well-being a priority every day. Again, you ain't gotta be perfect, just focused— and committed. It's about exercising discipline and holding ourselves accountable to practicing the principles. The more consistency we have, the more consistent benefits we experience. When it comes to applying the five Ps on the daily, it's all about having a sincere commitment to living this shit with purpose. These simple practices may seem basic (and they are), but drilling the healthy fundamentals over and over is what exercising our greatness is built on.

Being devoted to putting in the work to keep our mental health strong is really nonnegotiable. We simply cannot afford to not make mental and emotional wellness a priority in our lives. Staying hydrated and making mindful choices about nutrition are investments that are well worth it. What we choose to consume can either enslave and poison us and make us sick and diseased, or it can nourish and energize us, heal us, make us well, and help us thrive. Making good dietary decisions is a choice and an act of self-love and self-respect. Enjoying regular workout activities benefits the spirit and mind, not just the physique. When we sweat, we release physical and mental toxins, our mood is uplifted, and we can repurpose unproductive emotions in constructive ways. We need strength, flexibility, endurance, and vitality to live well, and exercise is one of the very best ways to develop those attributes in our character. If we don't exercise the greatness in our own bodies, our bodies will become burdens to bear instead of vehicles of vitality. Respecting rest and taking time to recharge regularly actually gives us more energy to work with. We grow when we rest. Sleep is not the cousin of death, sleep is the partner of life. Vocation without vacation is a violation, and it's just not sustainable. Even the seasons rest. We thrive when we do so as well.

Now, with all that being said, and we know that it is true, without consistency and discipline it's just not possible to reap the long-term benefits. These are the tools, but tools don't work unless we work them and continue to work them. We have to use the tools. There is no way around it; you may tell yourself you are not disciplined but you gonna have to stop saying that kind of counterproductive shit to yourself and believe that you can become the kind of person that is disciplined. We're gonna have to learn to override feelings that create excuses. You're going to have to reprogram your thoughts and feelings to support your well-being instead of entertaining too many thoughts and feelings that sabotage it. You're going to have to stay inspired in order to stay disciplined. We have to apply the behavioral science and trust the process and be relentless to make the kind of long-lasting changes that become automatic in your lifestyle.

Learning how to stay inspired and consistently take the actions that support well-being is the secret sauce that keeps all the mind-body benefits flowing and growing for the long haul. Knowing how to continuously inspire ourselves makes all the difference in the world.

This is why the five principles are truly a way of life.

Stay Inspired: The Power of Self-Talk

One of the ways I've learned to stay committed to my healthy lifestyle is to develop an understanding of how self-talk affects my ability to stay focused and inspired. When I commit to a mission, I've learned that my self-talk can either boost it or break it. When something is difficult for you, what's your self-talk like? When you say you're going to do something, and it gets hard, how do you speak to yourself?

Keeping your word with yourself is powerful and important. The words we say to ourselves matter. The vibrations of our words are real, and they have a real effect on matter. I ain't no botanist, but the legendary "peanut man" himself George Washington Carver said that speaking to plants with positive words of encouragement helps them grow, and I think as a scientist, an agriculturalist, a horticulturist, a chemurgist, an eco-visionary, a conservationist, and more, he knew a thing or two about it.

It's not only words. Music also has similar effects. The field of science that looks at the influences of sound waves and their effect on solid bodies is called sonochemistry. But you don't have to have a degree in science to know that the energy of words or music affects you. A well-intentioned compliment and a mean-spirited critique will definitely stimulate different chemical reactions and responses. An uplifting reggae song about giving thanks for life is gonna hit different than a trap drill song about killing opps and running through bitches. It just is. And we know this without a peer-reviewed study. Shit, *we* are the peer-reviewed study. The same way we know if we yell harsh, negative words at our kids it will affect them differently than if we speak to them calmly with words of encouragement, kindness, and love. We know because we know how those same options make us feel.

The power question is: How can we better use this knowledge in our own self-talk? How do what we say to ourselves and how we say it affect our ability to stay focused and consistent in our healthy life-style practices? The better we learn to appreciate that how we talk to ourselves plays a major role in how we live our lives, the better we can direct our lives in healthier ways. We have to learn to speak to ourselves like George Washington Carver spoke to his plants and flowers. We have to feed ourselves affirmations to be our best selves. We tell ourselves what we want to hear all the time. We believe all kinds of negative and limiting things about ourselves. Why can't we build a system of talking to ourselves that's gonna have a healthy effect in our lives?

THE HIP-HOP FLAVOR

A cheesy but enlightening study done by a Swiss cheese maker and a team of researchers from the Bern University of Arts looked at how different types of music—classical, rock, hip-hop, and more—affect the taste of cheese. The researchers put twenty-two-pound wheels of cheese in separate wooden crates in the cheese maker's cheese cellar. For six months, each cheese was exposed to a continuous, twenty-four-hour loop of one song using a device that transduced the sound waves directly into the cheese wheels. One was played music from Mozart, another exposed to Led Zeppelin, and another one was played "Jazz (We've Got)" by A Tribe Called Quest. A few other cheeses were exposed to other music and some to simple tones of particular frequencies, and one cheese was just aged in silence, as a control. In two rounds of blind taste-tests, culinary experts unanimously chose A Tribe Called Quest's cheese as the best and said it was "remarkably fruity, both in smell and taste, and significantly different from the other samples." The researchers are now exploring marketing cheese based on the music it was aged to.

Think—Feel—Become

> No problem can be solved from the same level of consciousness that created it.
>
> —*Albert Einstein*

In 1981 in New Hampshire, Harvard psychologist Ellen Langer and a team of researchers conducted a study on groups of seventy-to-eighty-year-old men. The study was conducted at a monastery in New Hampshire in two separate five-day retreats. The elders were split into two groups. After preliminary physicals, a series of biochemical measurements were taken and cognitive performance tests were given to the first group. They were then asked to pretend they were young again; to imagine they were actually twenty-two years younger than they were. They did activities that were as similar as possible to what they were doing back then. This was in 1981, so they were given all sorts of environmental nudges from 1959 to remind them of their younger selves: old newspapers, magazines, movies, and TV shows from that era, and they listened to songs that were popular on the radio at the time. They talked about what would have been "current topics" such as sports and political events that were happening at the time. All of the cues from that period were designed to help the elders fully go there in imagining the state of being they were in at the time.

The experiment with the first group ran for five days; the following week, the researchers brought the other group of elderly men to the retreat. As a control, these men were only instructed to *reminisce* about their lives of twenty-two years ago, but not to pretend they were younger. From both groups, before and after the experiment, the researchers took lots of measurements and compared them. The results were amazing.

The measurements showed that the bodies of both groups of men were physiologically younger, both in structure and in function. They noted changes and improvements in posture, joint flexibility, and arthritis symptoms, grip strength, eyesight, hearing, and even changes in height (due to better posture), weight loss, and even their walking gait. They took memory tests and showed improvement, and all scored better on cognitive tests—as much as 60 percent better. Based on the results, it's as if these guys *actually became younger* and this was only a five-day retreat! And dig this, the guys from the first group who had pretended they were younger showed significantly more change and improvements than the control group who only reminisced. The researcher reported that by the end of the study, she was playing touch football with some of the elders who had given up their canes as a result of the experiment.

That's powerful, right? Our ability to change is incredible. The retreat sparked the elders' mental circuits to fire like their younger selves would have, and like magic—no, better yet—like science, their body chemistry responded in real time. The change was mental *and* physical. If I could post a giant reminder on a huge billboard on every city around the world to drive the point home, it would say: *"We become what we constantly think about."*

What's Really Real?

You ever play that game as a kid in the car, when you try to see who can spot how many other cars of a certain color? I play that game with my youngest son. We'll decide we're looking for red cars and it's like all of a sudden, red cars seem like they're everywhere. Have you ever experienced that? It's like it's way easier to spot something when that's what we are looking for. We see what we expect to see. It's actually called "red-car syndrome," or sometimes it's also referred to as confirmation bias. It could be a word or just about anything. Once you expect something it feels like it happens everywhere you look. In reality, there's not necessarily an actual objective increase in occurrence. It's just that you've started to notice it because you expect to. That's why it's so easy to find an excuse if we don't really want to do something. Or for the same reason, why we're more likely to find a way to do something when that's what we are determined to do. We are literally hypnotized by the stories we tell ourselves over and over. We are hypnotized by whatever we repeatedly think and do, and what we do unconsciously in a suggestive state is that much more mesmerizing and impactful on our thoughts-and-feelings loop. As I mentioned earlier on, TV watching is one of the most powerful examples of how easily we fall into a hypnotic state without even realizing it. When you're into that show you're feeling every emotion the plot is "suggesting." You're in a state of trance that suspends reality and replaces it with what the show is guiding, inducing, and influencing you to accept as true in the moment.

You agree to "believe" it.

If you watch a scary movie, you know that it's fake and that you're sitting down to watch actors play out a script, but when Freddy Krueger jumps out on that screen your heart is beating the same way it would if Freddy Krueger was actually in front of your ass! On the emotional level, the brain and body don't separate what's real from what's imagined. If you believe it, even for pretend, once there's a real buy-in, your body responds as if it were real. If you tested your blood during a scary movie your body chemistry would reveal the same cortisol levels of fear as if you were going through the scenario yourself in real life. This is one of many reasons why I avoid watching negative drama play out on television over and over, and I even stopped listening to certain kinds of music with negative perspectives and vibes because I know it makes impressions and subconscious suggestions that are subliminally absorbed; and plus, I'm a Pisces and we just absorb shit different.

Thought Control

If we become what we constantly think about, what we believe to be true, how do we make the most of this in our lives? Experts have acknowledged that all hypnosis, on some level, is self-hypnosis.

Self-hypnosis involves preparing our mind and body to be receptive to suggestion, and then repeatedly reinforcing our desired intention. We can use this tool to consciously and consistently choose to focus, seed, and reprogram ourselves in ways that are fruitful to our well-being. We have to exercise our power to be selective with the thoughts we pay attention to and regulate how much focus we give the different thoughts. There's productive thinking and unproductive thinking. A high-quality thought is one that's uplifting and empowering and productive; it makes you feel confident, encouraged, and loved. A low-quality thought is unproductive and negative, fearful, critical, hurtful, or mean. As we find ourselves getting caught up in a low-quality thought pattern, the practice is to stop and replace it with a high-quality upgrade. That, my friend, is the self-mastery game in a nutshell. It's about exercising that "choice muscle" again and again. Some thoughts will be heavier than others but there ain't nothing we can't do if we learn to be skillful at managing our own thoughts. With the right attitude it ain't really shit that can stop us and it comes down to a choice: What kind of conversation with ourselves do we wanna entertain? Do we want to be our own worst critic or our own cornerman, coach, and encourager? If you don't root for you then how can you even expect to be successful? Are you going to root for you? Do you promise to have your own back? Then silence that negative stinking thinking, be more loving to yourself, be good to you, and speak to you with respect, compassion, and confidence. Tell yourself you can do it! Remind yourself that you are the kind of person that takes action. You have to train your own mind how to treat you. It's your right and responsibility. Exercise your right to program the mental atmosphere that you want in your own mind.

Let's come back to the emotional reactions we experience when we're really into a TV show or movie, or when we're deep into a book so much so that we forget about whatever else is happening around us. In this state, you're experiencing a hypnotic "trance" effect. This is a normal state of the mind that happens automatically when we are relaxed and fully engaged with our imagination. Self-hypnosis could be described as a kind of meditation with an intention or goal to consciously influence your own subconscious mind to replace an unwanted pattern of thoughts, emotions, or habits with new behaviors. If you don't vibe with the word hypnosis, just look at it as a technique for reinforcing an inner adjustment or mental shift you want to make. One of the most empowering feelings is to want to change and have the tools.

Self-Hypnosis: How to Practice

1. Prioritize time on your schedule to make your practice a regular thing. Find a comfortable spot to sit or lay down where you will be undisturbed for twenty to thirty minutes. Close your eyes and breathe slowly and deeply, in and out through your nose.

2. Use a hypnotic induction technique like soothing natural sounds or binaural beats coupled with the slow, deep breathing and muscle relaxing. Focus your awareness to recognize and release any and all tense areas in your body.

3. Introduce a suggestion and repeat and visualize it throughout the session. Use simple and clear statements to seed yourself with new thoughts, ideas, actions, responses, or behaviors that you intend to do differently—for example, when facing a challenge, or how you may want to think or feel differently about yourself or some situation or circumstance. People use self-hypnosis to support and reinforce all sorts of lifestyle changes, from behavior changes like quitting smoking or having a better relationship with food, to dealing with psych issues like anxiety, anger management, or improving self-esteem and self-confidence. Self-suggestions phrased in the positive, present tense are called affirmations. Affirmations can focus

on any area of behavior that you intend to make a lasting psychological shift. "I am..." statements are great ways to phrase your affirmations. Some examples:

- I am calm under pressure.
- I am able to learn new things with joy and ease.
- I choose healthy options when I eat.
- I am consistently active and fit.
- I am respectful of rest and relaxation.
- I am worthy of a healthy life.
- I am disciplined and determined to maintain my wellness.
- I do what it takes to change my life.

4. After you've repeated your affirmations for the duration of your session, you can transition yourself back into your normal alert state by slowly counting from ten down to one. Open your eyes, wiggle your fingers and toes, stretch out your arms and legs, give thanks, and go on with your day.

Remember, the emotional conviction of your intention and the volume of repetitions of your affirmations are what help them take root in the subconscious. With consistent practice you will learn to enter a state of trance more quickly. If you're not sure about trying self-hypnosis on your own, you can find plenty of guided recordings online. A few books to check out for more in-depth insight and research on self-hypnosis and auto suggestion practices are *You are the Placebo* by Dr. Joe Dispenza, Ra Un Nefer Amen's classic, *Stress Free for Life*, *Close Your Eyes, Get Free* by Grace Smith, and *Instant Self-Hypnosis* by Forbes Robbins Blair.

NOTHING WILL WORK UNLESS YOU DO.

—MAYA ANGELOU

Consistency: The Rhythm of Discipline

> If you don't have the mental capacity to be that obsessed about what you're trying to get . . . then motherfucker you ain't never gonna have it.
>
> —*C. T. Fletcher, the Compton*
> *Superman, body builder*

Consistency means doing something continuously, repeatedly, persistently, reliably, regularly, routinely, and relentlessly. Let's immediately debunk the myth that consistency is hard. Consistency is not hard. Consistency is automatic. In fact, the law of consistency is always at work. The power of consistency is already at work in your life right now, every day. Not just in obvious functions like your heartbeat, your breathing, or blinking. Whatever you're consistently doing is expressing the law of consistency. The kicker is this: that's what's producing the results you're experiencing. Human beings are habitual creatures. We constantly do the same things over and over again. We have all sorts of routines that we do. Some we are conscious of and other habits happen subconsciously. A chain-smoker is consistent with smoking. A TV watcher is consistent in binging on their favorite shows. Many of us entertain our fears and negative thoughts without fail on a regular basis. People sometimes say it's their lack of consistency that explains why they don't achieve certain positive habits in their life. But there's no lack of consistency. Lack of consistency is not the issue in our lives because we are all consistent every day, in many things.

Our Patterns Are Powerful

The question is, what are we choosing to be consistent in and why? Why are we so consistent in finding excuses instead of taking actions in our best interest? Why are we so consistent in eating things we know are not healthy? Why are we constantly skipping exercise? Why do we consistently feel tired? Why are we consistently inconsistent? Is it because we naturally choose to be consistent in what we enjoy, or what is easy and comfortable? Is the comfort zone a home that nourishes growth and well-being, or is the comfort zone a prison that we hide behind the bars of excuses in, reinforcing unskillful habits and unproductive thinking? Are we committed to complacency and calling it a comfort zone? Going for a morning run would be exhilarating, but lying in bed scrolling on the phone is easier. Drinking water is good for me but drinking this root beer seems more satisfying. Indulging in the things we enjoy that might not be the absolute best is fine at times—that's the spice of life. But balance is key. We can acquire a taste for discipline, too.

Eliminate Excuses

Excuses are like spiderwebs to a fly. Once you get tangled up in them, it's over. Consistency is natural and automatic; excuses are what make it hard to stay consistent. Like opinions, everyone has excuses, but our excuses can be like invisible bars that keep us from implementing real changes for the better in our lives. Sometimes there are circumstances beyond our control that we have to adjust to and recalibrate our expectations, that's real. But if we notice, not always but surely most of the time, if we really wanna do something, we find workarounds so that excuses don't stop us.

In terms of winning the battle of constructive self-talk over negative patterns and excuses that keep us from sticking to the positive changes we commit to, we need to create a consistent practice where we are focusing on the thoughts, feelings, actions, and habits we want to embody. Discipline is about cultivating a stick-to-the-mission mentality: What's the mission? Let's go! It's about identifying and eliminating our tendency to justify excuses. It's cultivating a let-nothing-stop-you kind of spirit.

Consistent discipline is like a force of nature; it wields its own influence over circumstances and helps us shape our reality like a blacksmith forging his own sword. It's how we keep ourselves sharp. It's what empowers us to know that, step by step, anything is possible. Discipline is the rent you pay on the life you want to live.

But I know sometimes the word discipline is a put-off to some people. So, pulling from my musical background, let's look at discipline as a form of having "rhythm."

Ride the Rhythm

> Success or greatness comes with a roller-coaster ride, anybody can apply the marathon concept to what they do.
>
> —*Nipsey Hussle*

When you're incorporating a steady pattern of discipline in your life, you are living with rhythm and that's when you start to feel like you're finding your groove. Rhythmic *entrainment* is the technical term for the synchronization that happens when we're listening to music and we automatically start bobbing our heads, tapping our feet, clapping our hands, or snapping our fingers to the rhythm. We perceive the pattern and if we dig it, we instinctively move in sync with it. When we perceive rhythmic patterns in music, they can influence the creation of different emotional states. Entrainment is the adjustment, influence, or moderation of one behavior either to synchronize or to be in rhythm with another behavior. In short, rhythm stimulates rhythm.

Rhythm is extremely important in everything we do. Rhythm influences the frequencies and states of the brain, it's present in the steady beating of the heart and the continuous blood flow, the breathing in and out of oxygen, sleeping and waking cycles, the menstrual cycle, and even the balancing act of walking or running. Rhythm governs time itself. Bodily rhythms are indicators of health or illness. When a physician checks the internal rhythms of a patient's heart, blood pressure, and pulse they are looking for irregularities in these rhythms to determine risk factors and diagnose symptoms.

Living with consistent discipline and regular practices is akin to having a good sense of musical rhythm. By establishing a rhythm of discipline in our lives through routine and repetition, we set ourselves up to take advantage of the momentum of entrainment to bring order and harmony to our lives. Instead of seeing consistency as monotonous and boring, we can reframe it and see it as having a rhythmic lifestyle. The drumbeat and the heartbeat are not-so-distant cousins. When we get our lives moving in a meaningful cadence, life is more manageable.

Broken Rhythms

There are natural breaks in rhythm; it's not all about nonstop, go, go, go. Rhythm involves certain actions and certain rests, at regular intervals. Rhythm is never static. We all experience changes and challenges, but if we've established a strong, consistent groove in our norm, the easier we can get back in step or adapt and improvise accordingly.

In ancient times, living with the rhythms of nature was the norm. Today, with technological advancements and modern conveniences, society has gotten out of sync with these natural rhythms. But the more we coordinate our activities with the natural flow of our recurring days, weeks, months, and years, the more alignment we feel with the flow of nature.

A daily routine can help minimize stress, keep you on track, and help you and your whole family live a more balanced and productive life. Our schedules, routines, and rituals set the tones, beats, and grooves of our lives. When we feel like things are chaotic and disorganized or not quite falling into place, routines can help us reestablish and feel more of a sense of order.

Consistency with the five Ps is about making a solid agreement with yourself to do your best to stick to the healthy habits and lifestyle that you want. By creating a structure and putting systems and schedules in place, you create a standard to hold yourself accountable to and you know when you are getting too far off track so you can make the necessary adjustments. If surprises pop up, no prob; because you have a healthy norm established, you won't get lost in the sauce because you know that you can handle the variables and snap right back into your flow. No two days are going to go exactly the same. No plan is going to always flow exactly as planned. We have to learn how to dance with life as it comes and that's why we need to have a good sense of rhythm, so that even when things throw us off, we can always lock back into the groove and not miss a beat. Don't let the term discipline intimidate you—just keep doing your dance.

Pimp the System

> Know what you want. Don't worry about the reward;
> just set in motion the machinery to achieve it.
>
> —*Bruce Lee*

Whereas specific goals provide a direction and a target to aim for, it's actually your *process*, the system or systems you follow, that makes it happen or not. Committing to and trusting the process is most important. Living in accordance with good systems in place is what makes a healthy lifestyle sustainable for the long haul.

In his best-selling book, *Atomic Habits*, James Clear breaks it down like this: "Goals are good for planning your progress and systems are good for actually making progress. Goals can provide direction and even push you forward in the short-term, but eventually a well-designed system will always win. Having a system is what matters. Committing to the process is what makes the difference."

Goals define what we want to achieve, but systems create the ongoing lifestyle habits that produce and sustain the results. Your goal might be to become a meditator. You could systematize that goal by committing to waking up at 7:00 a.m. for the next thirty days, Monday through Friday, to practice meditating for ten minutes. Your commitment to your process is the system you put in place, and the results will naturally come out of committing to the system. You become a meditator by sticking to the system. In fact, the journey is the destination; the system is the goal itself. So, when it comes to achieving and maintaining your healthy lifestyle habits, build and work your system and the rest will follow.

CALM UNDER PRESSURE

For five consecutive days, try this five-minute exercise. Play rain sounds and chant, "I am calm under pressure" (or any desired trait you wish to acquire) as part of your morning and evening rituals. Notice how this can influence you as you move through challenging circumstances.

Mission Mode: Staying Inspired

Power means work overtime scientifically, so if I put
in work, over time, I know it's meant for me.
—*Stic, "Put in the Work"*

Consistency is a physical act but a mental art. The pattern of consistency in the mind will be expressed in the actions of our lives, and in the same way, as we take consistent action, even if we don't always feel like it, those actions will shift our perspectives of ourselves. It's a conscious and mindful choice we make moment by moment. We have to train our beliefs just like we train anything else. Self-hypnosis might seem like hocus-pocus on the surface but it's rooted in real insight on how behavior works. It's nothing more than a practice of putting yourself in a receptive state of mind and coaching yourself to embody the perspective you want to live your life through. It's learning how to effectively be your own coach. Consistency is being rich in *ritual*.

When we are relentless, we are incessant, not easily stopped, determined, committed, resolute, and steadfast. This isn't to be confused with stubbornness—'cause you do wanna be flexible and not rigid. Consistency is about having a relentless attitude to persevere, a conviction that detours will not deter your determination—that unstoppable spirit of doing what needs to be done, like clockwork, and appreciating the process, whatever it takes, over and over and over. Wherever I see the character trait of relentlessness of consistency, I salute it. Nature is relentless. Life is relentless. Time is relentless. The heart is relentless. The breath is relentless. It's that "if you fall, still get up, no let up" type of shit.

"Keep Going" Is the Mantra

We ain't gonna meditate for one day and expect to master the practice in one sitting. You don't read one book and instantly become an expert on a subject. Skills take time and regular practice to develop. You wouldn't eat one salad and expect to lose weight, nor would you expect to eat a lot of calories in one day and expect immediate weight gain. You don't hit the gym one day and expect to get strong right away. You don't stretch one time and expect to be flexible like a rubber band. You don't take one day off a year from the grind and expect to feel energized, rested, and recharged the other 364 days.

To achieve more clarity and peace of mind, we need to be consistent in our meditation and mindfulness practices. To be nourished nutritionally, we have to be consistently choosing nutritious things over toxic things, eating well, and staying hydrated. To have strength, flexibility, energy, and endurance we have to consistently exercise those attributes. To feel rested, relaxed, and rejuvenated we have to consistently take the time to replenish, relax, and recharge. The key ingredient in developing and maintaining all of these healthy qualities is building systems of consistency in our lives.

Curate your Power Zone: Appreciation, Gratitude, and Celebration

The comfort zone is cool but let me introduce you to the power zone. Your comfort zone keeps you cozy in complacency, but your power zone is curated to inspire, motivate, and encourage you on an everyday basis.

Power Zone Toolbox—What Inspires You?

Curating your power zone means identifying what inspires you and literally building your own kit of reliable tools that help you stay motivated and inspired. Your kit can include whatever you like, but be specific. Name the song, album, person, film, scene, magazine, book, activity, place, time of day—get granular with it. You're identifying and assembling a powerful list of people, places, and things that you resonate with in a deep way and draw inspiration from. Having your own curated power-zone list is a game changer in staying inspired and consistent. Take the time to consciously collect or connect with those sources and keep them handy so you can access them on a regular basis.

Gratitude Attitude

We've established that if you want your body to do something consistently, your mind has to affirm it consistently. What feeds your spirit? Appreciate and celebrate it! I believe a gratitude attitude is the key to consistent inspiration. When you ain't feeling particularly motivated, find something to be grateful for, celebrate it, and watch what happens. Even the smallest things count. Celebration means showing appreciation with enthusiasm; to recognize, affirm, salute, and express gratitude for the impactful people, places, moments, events, lessons, ideas, art, knowledge, nature, experiences, achievements, and realizations of our lives. Imagine living every day in celebration of what inspires you. Imagine choosing what you give your time, energy, and attention to, at least for a part of each day, with the intention of supporting your well-being. What if you dedicated yourself to curating what moves you so that you're constantly and intentionally having experiences that lift your spirit and keep you focused on what supports your best life? What if you intentionally curate your tools and create regimens, rituals, and routines that reinforce your well-being? Guarantee you wouldn't regret it.

What makes things last? Appreciating them and taking care of them. What makes love last? Appreciation. What makes us keep our commitments? Continuing to appreciate why we are committed in the first place. If we're celebrating what moves us every day and every way, there'll be no limit to inspiration. Practicing the five Ps consistently is an investment that will continue to appreciate throughout your life, because what we appreciate in our lives *appreciates* in our lives.

Keep going is the mantra!

Strive for the Five: Five Creative Ways to Apply the Five Ps in Everyday Life

All this shit is customizable; you can put it together in a way that works for you. Here are five ways to spark your own creative ideas for further implementing the five Ps in your day to day.

1. Power Up Your Birthday with the Five P's

Back in the day, I used to celebrate my birthday by getting as drunk and high as I could and eating a bunch of unhealthy, sugary shit. I've since learned that birthdays are about celebrating life and vitality instead. So, on my birthdays I've learned to try and practice healthy activities that allow me to show my appreciation for my health and vitality!

Instead of your usual celebration, try this fun and healthy twist instead.

MINDSET. Do a mindfulness practice like meditation, read something interesting, take a class and learn something new, try a new skill, or teach someone something you know.

NUTRITION. Eat and drink something nutritionally powerful. Even if you do engage in some indulgences, make sure to also, even if just symbolically, give a nod to your nutritional health. Have a shot of wheatgrass. Drink a gallon of water. Eat your favorite healthy foods. If you usually drink and/or smoke, try a new ritual of abstaining on your b-day.

EXERCISE. Get a birthday workout in! Do a number of push-ups matching your age. Go for a run. Hit the gym. Do a yoga session. Go for a walk or a bike ride or rock climbing. Ain't no sweat like birthday sweat! You will feel like you've given yourself a great gift.

REST. Hit the steam room or sauna. Sleep in if you can. Plan in advance to be off work if you are able. Take a relaxing hot bath or shower. Take a nap outside. Go be by some water. Schedule a pedicure or massage. Treat yourself to some spa services.

CONSISTENCY. Do something that inspires you. See a movie. Go to a concert. Visit a museum. Go to a boxing event. Go out dancing. Arrange a photoshoot for yourself. Be generous to the homeless. Volunteer for a cause you believe in. Create some form of art or music or build something with your hands. Listen to an inspiring motivational speaker. Go to church or kick it with your homies.

And shit, if you want to eat three scoops of vegan ice cream instead on your b-day—do it! Don't beat yourself up about it—it's your day, enjoy it!

2. Master the Morning with the Five P's

Morning routines are well researched for their benefits, and healthy, productive, and successful people from all walks of life thrive by them. Getting up early and greeting your day with a powerful routine before the challenges of the day get in the way will set a powerful tone and create positive ripple effects in your life. As the Yoruba saying goes, the master of the morning is the owner of the day.

Here's a flow inspired by the five Ps you can try for your morning routine:

Meditate: Ten minutes

Activate: Do fifty reps or five sets of ten of any calisthenics exercise you choose

Energize: Drink a cup of warm water, some tea, or a smoothie, and/or eat a breakfast that consists of a carb (like fruit, oatmeal, toast, or some other healthy carb), a protein of your choice, a green, and a healthy fat (like avocado, olives, or nut butter).

Elevate: Pray, read or watch something inspiring, or write in your gratitude journal for five minutes.

Enterprise: Take ten minutes or more to determine the three most productive things you need to do as far as your work or personal goals and do those three things first.

The late, great distance runner, weight lifter, and spiritual teacher Sri Chinmoy once said, "In the morning if we can energize ourselves with physical activities, then we can accomplish so many things during the rest of the day. That is why I say sports and physical fitness are of supreme importance. If we neglect the physical and let the body become weak, then the mind also becomes weak."

If you can devote anywhere from twenty to thirty minutes to an hour of your morning to investing in yourself like this, if not daily then at least a few times a week, you're going to feel incredibly inspired.

3. Mantra Your Five P's

Here are some mantras you can memorize and use as affirmations during your positive self-talk practices:

My mind is at peace.
I hydrate and eat to thrive.
I exercise for strength, flexibility, endurance, and vitality.
I respect rest and have fun.
I take consistent actions that support well-being.
I stay inspired.

Action Mantra:

Feel like it or not
I take action

'cause the law of action
makes good things happen.

Seeds Mantra:

The actions I take
from the moment I awake
set the tone of my day and the life I create.
The choices I make
in the moments each day
are the seeds that develop the life I create.

4. Five-Minute Movement

If you don't have a lot of time in the day to train, here is an easy, effective go-to routine to keep in your toolbox. Rest for one minute in between each exercise:

One minute of jumping jacks
One minute of squats
One minute of sit-ups
One minute of push-ups
One-minute plank

Do as many of each as you can within each minute.

5. Five P's Weekly Challenge

This is an easy way to integrate elements of the five Ps throughout the week:

- Meditate on Mondays.
- Eat healthy on Tuesdays.

- Drink a gallon of water on Wednesdays.
- Do something restorative on Thursdays.
- Do something inspiring on Fridays.

The Law of Consistency

I want to leave you with one last thing. Whether we're putting in the work or you don't, either way, we're being consistent. The real "aha" is applying the law of consistency toward a healthy outcome. Enhancing vitality gives us greater capacity to handle our lives—mentally, physically, and spiritually. More chi! More life. More resilience. I have learned to respect the law of consistency as a superpower. Not only in terms of my well-being practices, but in general; it's just a part of how I'm built. I've been rapping since fifth grade, and I might sit my pen down from time to time to breathe life in a different way, but after all this time I'm still emceeing. I'm a long-distance runner. I keep going. Consistency is something I strive to live, breathe, and practice. Now, that don't mean I don't still have plenty of things that I aim to be more consistent with, because I definitely do. But what I know fasho, is that consistency is more than a notion to me; it's a fundamental value that I respect and aspire to embody in my words, actions, relationships, and lifestyle.

Consistency generates its own energy. Once it clicks, and you make the connection with the power of consistency, it's on! Discovering a new source of energy inspires you to work with it to understand it more and make use of it in your life. Second by second, eons accumulate. Drop by drop, water erodes the rock. When you take consistent action toward something you value or want to achieve, no matter if you always feel like it or not, the results manifest. The law of consistent action causes a chain reaction. It's just a matter of time.

Bonus Inspo

A list of books and films that inspired the
songs on my *Workout II* album:

Let's Go Champ—*The Charge* by Brendon Burchard, *Mindful Athlete* by George Mumford, *Coaching and Mentoring for Success* by Jane Smith, *Sports Psychology for Dummies, As a Man Thinketh* by James Allen

Put in the Work—*The Power of Habit* by Charles Duhigg, *The Obstacle Is the Way* by Ryan Holiday, *The Personal MBA* by Josh Kaufman, *Soar* by T. D. Jakes, *Work Clean* by Dan Charnas, *Complete Family Wealth* by James E. Hughes

Motivated—*Transformed* by Remi Adeleke, *Can't Hurt Me* by David Goggins, *The Art of War* by Sun Tzu, *The Warrior Ethos* by Steven Pressfield, *The Science of Motivation* by Brian Tracy

Goal Medalist—*The Greatest: The Haile Gebrselassie Story* by Jim Denison, *The Code of the Extraordinary Mind* by Vishen Lakhiani, *Float Like a Butterfly* (film)

Uplifting—*Eat Plants Lift Iron* by Stic of dead prez and Afya Ibomu, *Sport and Meditation* by Sri Chinmoy, *The Black Prince* by Robby Robinson, *C. T. Fletcher: My Magnificent Obsession* (film)

Run—*Sprinter* (film), *Born to Run* by Christopher McDougall, *Run for Your Life* by Lopez Lomong, *4 Minute Mile* (film)

Me Time—*The Autobiography of Gucci Mane, Long Walk to Freedom* by Nelson Mandela

Stay Ready—*The Nature Fix* by Florence Williams, *The Way of the SEAL* by Mark Divine, *More Fire: How to Run the Kenyan Way* by Toby Tanser

Drink Water—*Your Body's Many Cries for Water* by Fereydoon Batmanghelidj, *The Hidden Messages in Water* by Masaru Emoto

Trust the Universe—*I Ching, Tao Te Ching* by Lao Tzu, *What the Buddha Taught* by Walpola Rahula Thero, *Astrophysics for People in a Hurry* by Neil deGrasse Tyson, *The Seven Spiritual Laws of Success* by Deepak Chopra, *Power vs. Force* by David R. Hawkins, *Kybalion* by Three Initiates, *The Art of Peace* by Morihei Ueshiba, translated by John Stevens

Qigong—*Qi Gong Healing Prescriptions* by Ra Un Nefer Amen

White Belt—*Striking Thoughts* by Bruce Lee, *Body Mind Mastery* by Dan Millman, *The Warrior Within* by John Little, *Tao of Jeet Kune Do* by Bruce Lee

Triumphant—*Muhammad Ali in His Own Words*, *The School of Greatness* by Lewis Howes, *Iron Ambition* by Mike Tyson

Raise the Bar—*Smarter Faster Better* by Charles Duhigg, *Atomic Habits* by James Clear, *The Possibility Principle* by Mel Schwartz

Acknowledgments

Completing this book was a marathon of the mind and spirit. I've learned, grown, and experienced so much in the process.

I give thanks to my team for helping bring it all into being.

To Afya, thank you for the epic journey together and the inspiring healthy lifestyle example you've shown me throughout the years. More health, life, and prosperity.

To my literary agent, Regina Brooks of Serendipity Literary Agency, you are the best at what you do! To Kelly, thanks for all your encouraging assistance with the writing process.

To my publisher, Hatchette Book Group/Balance—Nana, thank you for seeing and believing in the vision and value of the 5 P's and for extending such a supportive opportunity for me to share my journey.

To my feedback squad—my homies "D," Zayd, Nym, Shiek, Ken, Pree, Young Noble, and Martin Luther—thank you for listening and lending your thoughts, feedback, and encouragement throughout the process.

This labor of love would not be complete without you all.

Index

About the Author

Khnum "Stic" Ibomu—widely known as Stic from the legendary hip-hop group dead prez and founder of RBG FIT CLUB—is an award-winning hip-hop artist and producer, certified long-distance running coach, and an adjunct professor at the Clive Davis Institute at New York University. Dubbed "the father of fit-hop," Stic pioneered the fit-hop music genre with his groundbreaking albums *The Workout* and *Workout II*. His music and lifestyle have inspired millions around the world in personal growth and healthy living. Follow him on Instagram @stic.

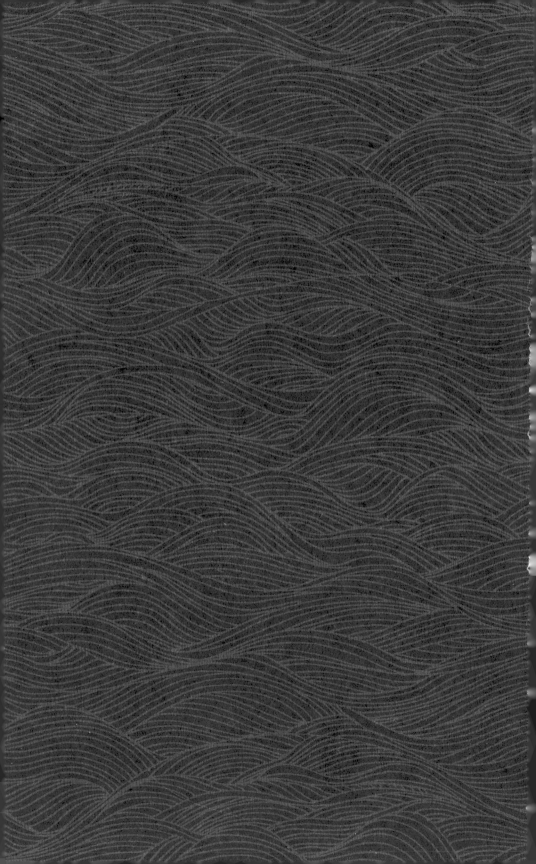